A Pink Ribbon Journey

Wendy Clarke

authorHOUSE®

AuthorHouse™
1663 Liberty Drive
Bloomington, IN 47403
www.authorhouse.com
Phone: 1-800-839-8640

Published by AuthorHouse   07/17/2012

ISBN: 978-1-4634-3619-3 (sc)
ISBN: 978-1-4634-3617-9 (hc)
ISBN: 978-1-4634-3618-6 (e)

This book is dedicated to the memory of all the courageous women that have been taken far too soon by breast cancer and to every sister that has experienced the ravages of cancer and cancer treatment.

Dear Survivor,

Please accept my invitation to come along with me on my personal journey through breast cancer and treatment. Allow me to share with you how God carried me through the worst experience of my life and strengthened my faith. This book has been written for you. Your experience is unique and you are the only one that knows how you feel. I pray this book gives you what God needs you to have. As you read about all my experiences through breast cancer and treatment, I hope you have the sense that you are not alone on your journey. Through these pages, I hope you laugh, cry, and allow your spirit to be calmed. Breast cancer is a roller coaster ride full of surprises at every turn, but God is with you every second of every day. Although I do not know you, I know you are there going through your own struggles. My prayers are with you. We are part of a sisterhood of survivors praying for each other and growing stronger every day.

God bless our sisterhood,
Wendy Clarke

Introduction

*All the world's a stage, and the men
And women merely players... William Shakespeare*

*B*ear with me while I attempt to share with you the worst time of my life. My story is not brilliant, nor spectacular, but for some familiar or new. I am no one special and have not done anything extraordinary. Apart from being a breast cancer survivor, I am a child of God with a story to tell. I am a middle-aged woman, two times married with three children I adore and cherish. I have two handsome sons and one beautiful daughter. My husband, Randal is a handsome man of 50. He works for a local towing company as a tow truck operator. He works hard and is better at his job than any of those twenty somethings. My oldest son, Nicholas, or Nick as he prefers, is 22 and a successful journeyman mechanic. My younger son, Matthew, or Matt as he prefers, is 19 and is well on his way climbing the corporate ladder at a national bank. My princess, Melissa is sweet sixteen and has a great knack for juggling school, work, friends, boys and more boys. My mom, Delilah, is a spry 84 years of age and has been my best friend my entire life. My father, Norman, died in 1997 from leukemia, a profound loss for my family and myself. I have two older brothers, Terry and Bryan. Both are happily married with families of their own. I have one sister, Linda, residing in Seattle, Washington.

As for me, I am 44 years of age and can clearly remember when 44 seemed like a lifetime away. Now it is upon me and threatening 45 very soon. I have worked a few different professions through the years. When I was married to my first husband early in our marriage I worked at a care home for elderly women. When my children were small, I taught myself to sew and had my own children's clothing company. When my first marriage ended, I went to university and received my Bachelor of Arts Degree with a major in English. After graduation, I tutored ESL students before my family and I moved to South Korea. While living in Korea, Randal and I both taught English while home schooling our own kids. Upon our return to Canada, I briefly taught ESL in Victoria, British Columbia. Due to a lack of employment for Randal, we decided to pack up and move to where the jobs were plentiful. We now reside in northern Canada, Fort St. John, British Columbia. Well, that is the quick and easy about my family and me.

Oh! I almost forgot to give honourable mention to some other very important family members, our three cherished cats. All three are delightful in their own way. My cat Mia is four years old, and is an adorable kitten size calico. She is very possessive of me and takes excellent care of me. Mia's best friend is my daughter's cat, Teddy. Teddy is also four years old and of average size. He has beautiful blonde fur and the most incredible green eyes. Finally, we have our Tiger Lily. Tiger Lily is three years old. She has a pretty face crowning her rather obese body, but she is ours and we love her.

Life Before Breast Cancer

Come to me, all you who are weary
and burdened, and I will give you
rest. Take my yoke upon you and
learn from me, for I am gentle and
humble in heart and you will find
rest for your souls. (Matthew 11:28-29)

Before I was diagnosed with breast cancer, my life had been spiralling out of control. I had numerous problems and issues, which resulted in a deep depression and a unhealthy serving of anxiety. The holiday season of 2007 had culminated into one of the most depressing, confusing and desperate times of my life. This Christmas season was even worse than the Christmas when my father was dying and the Christmas my daughter was born.

Please do not misunderstand. Giving birth to my daughter was an answer to a lifelong prayer, but her arrival into this world was a frightening and uncertain experience. She was born with a rare condition that seriously threatened her life. She was born with a diaphragmatic hernia. At some point during the pregnancy, her bowel had moved up through her diaphragm and into her left lung cavity. The doctors did not even know if she had a left lung. She was given a 20% chance of surviving, and was immediately air lifted to the B.C. Children's Hospital in Vancouver. Her father and I were both shocked and terrified. I was dumbfounded as to why God would give me the daughter I prayed for so much and then just take her away, but God did something amazing for me that I will never forget.

As two female nurses were wheeling me from the recovery room to a private room, I pulled the blanket over my head wishing the world would end. As I did so I heard a masculine voice inside my head say," Don't worry. She's going to be okay." I knew I was given divine comfort, and I hung onto those words until the day she came home all put back together. Through this experience people offered me all the usual kind of clichés, "God never gives you more than you can handle." "What doesn't kill you makes you stronger." "Yada, yada, yada." The only words that helped me through this nightmare were the words I had heard in my head. Obviously, Melissa is a healthy girl today and has not had any health issues since. As tough as that Christmas season was, and the Christmas season of 1997 when I watched my father die from leukemia, this Christmas season was my most desperate, and in many ways my most depressing.

Depression is one of the worst realities of the human experience. Depression can cripple a person's life and can destroy families. My depression was no different. My spirit had become crippled to the point I no longer knew who I was, or who I was supposed to be. My family and my life were falling apart before my very eyes, and I was helpless to do anything about it. During my depression, I prayed often throughout each day for some kind of help. All my problems and issues grew larger and larger as each day passed. I was beyond feeling overwhelmed. I was hopeless and desperate.

The first major problem in my life was my job. I worked at a care home as a residential care worker. The clients I served were developmentally challenged, and they were great. What special and wonderful people they were, and I enjoyed working with them. Often they would surprise me by how smart they really were. They taught me much in their own unique ways. My duties included personal hygiene, cooking, housekeeping, laundry, administering medications, and computer work. Sometimes it seemed like such a thankless job, but whenever I felt this way, I would remember ***Matthew 25:40 "I tell you the truth, whatever you did for one of the least of these brothers of mine you did for me."***

This job was an excellent way to serve God. The clients were wonderful people, the wages were good, and the benefits were great as well. Sounds like a great job, but there were numerous problems with this job. In reality, this job was less about serving the clients and more about surviving the never-ending negative politics between staff members and at times, management. Bad politics almost always start at the top and trickle all the way down to the bottom. There really were some excellent coworkers I enjoyed working with, but the majority of the staff were brutal to each other. The atmosphere of the job was one of fear and paranoia. I allowed this job to take over my entire life. All the fear and paranoia I experienced at work followed me home every day. I was exhausted after each shift and all I could do was sleep when I got home.

The most stressful part of my life was the most important part of my life. Like many depressed women, my marriage was in a state of chaos. For three years, I had been broken-hearted about my marriage. It was like watching a train wreck in slow motion. Randal and I had numerous issues between us and a great lack of communication. Like so many couples, we started out so well. We both had a great deal of respect for each other and treated each other like gold. It was terribly heartbreaking for me to accept the fact that we had gone from such happiness to such deep resentments.

Meeting Randal was one of the most exciting times of my life. I was like a lovesick teenager all over again. The butterflies would flutter about in my stomach whenever he was near. He reminded me of my father in many ways, but what really attracted me to him was his sense of humour. I relished his ability to make me laugh, and that made me feel like the world was not as scary as I thought it to be. Randal had made me his priority and made sure everyone knew it. He was everything I had wanted in a husband, and when he asked me to marry him I was over the moon. I was the happiest I had been in years.

The best part of being married to Randal was he had never been married before and had no children of his own. I am no fool. Randal was 40 years of age when we met and I knew he had other women in his past, but I was the chosen one. I was the one he wanted to be his wife, and that made me feel very special. We had many things in common and we both shared a sense of adventure. We were good for each other; each one concerned about the other. I would easily get lost in his big blue eyes and his face would delight me. Every night when we were in bed knowing he was beside me gave me a great sense of security and it was my favourite place in the whole world.

We had evolved from a happily married couple that had great respect for each other into two people that were no more than roommates, no longer getting along and seemingly hating one another. We had grown so far apart and no longer had healthy, open communication. In fact, we no longer had any communication left at all. For a significant period, we did not even share the same bed, and this made me feel extremely lonely and rejected. The place I had felt most secure and my favourite place in the whole world was gone. I still loved my husband too much to give up and I prayed for my marriage all the time. I missed my best friend desperately and wanted him back.

Marriage is a two way street and I played an equal role in our stagnant marriage. One big mistake I made was allowing the stress, fear, and paranoia of my job to come between Randal and me. I allowed my job to affect all aspects of my life and all my relationships. Another mistake I made was spending money. Whenever I felt hurt, lonely, rejected and abandoned I bought "stuff" hoping it would make me feel better, and it did - temporarily. All it really did was cause us financial troubles and added to the already existing resentments. Another cause to my strained marriage was my low self-esteem, or no self-esteem. I had lost all self-confidence I once had. The combination of a stressful job, failing marriage, financial troubles, low self-esteem and lack of self-confidence all added up to depression and anxiety. My depression and anxiety turned me into a hateful, resentful, suspicious and fearful woman no one knew anymore.

My depression affected everyone. It hurt Randal, the kids and my relationships with my mother and my mother in law. I know there were times when I treated my mom as if she was nothing but a nuisance. I often made her feel like I was too busy to be bothered with her. She had moved from Vancouver Island to Fort St. John to be close to her grandchildren and me. I am ashamed I made my mom feel like that after all the good and helpful things she has done for me. The other woman I ignored was Randal's mom, Lydia. I had stopped phoning her and months went by without any communication. Lydia has always treated me like a daughter, and she too has done many good and helpful things for me. I am also ashamed that I ignored her the way I did. I love Lydia very much and although no one could ever take the place of my own mom, she comes as close as anyone could ever get. I love you Mom, I love you Lydia, and I am sorry for treating you both as I did.

For a significant period of time I was genuinely oblivious to the fact that I was depressed. I knew something was wrong with my life and I knew there was something wrong with me both physically and mentally. I had no energy and was only capable of performing my duties at work. While at home, I was far too exhausted to do anything. When I came home from work all I could do was either sleep or sit and watch television. I did not live life; I merely went through the motions of living day after day.

I prayed all the time for change. Weeks would pass and nothing would change. I continued to pray and months would pass, and still no change. Still I prayed, and years passed with no change. I was at a complete loss at how to help myself, so I did nothing. Eventually my depression caused me to experience some crippling symptoms.

Every morning when I woke up, I felt a disturbing sensation encompass my entire body. It began in my heart and spread out from there. I immediately regretted waking up. I felt anger and resentment at the inevitability that there is always another day to live after the one I just got through. I would lie in bed and worry about all my problems. I would hope this new day would bring me something I could be happy about. I also hoped for some kind of resolution to at least one of my problems, but nothing. I prayed for some guidance as to how I could help myself. Again, nothing.

Another symptom of my depression that was equally disturbing would follow me throughout the entire day. This symptom physically hurt and was accompanied by a profound sense of hopelessness. I could feel a ball in my gut. This ball was engorged with fear, insecurity and self hatred. This feeling was always strong and it often made me feel like I could lose my sanity at any point. At times, I wished this enormity of fear and anxiety would just kill me, instead of torturing me every day. Trying to deal with the depression and its symptoms was exhausting. Whenever I could not stand to feel them, I ate comfort food. This remedy only caused me to gain weight causing more depression and prolonged my agony - truly a terrible coping mechanism.

My spirit found a new way to cope with my depression, so began my fear/denial pattern. Whenever my problems became too much for me to deal with I denied their existence. I would tell myself, "It's not as bad as I believe it is," or "I'm making something big out of nothing." Sometimes I would think about other people I knew and compared their problems to mine. I would convince myself their problems were much more serious than mine. I would also think about people around the world that suffer through war, starvation, illness, rape and poverty. I was able to realize that I had life good and denied I had any problems or issues. Gradually my fear/denial pattern began to deteriorate and its effectiveness was non - existent. My depression was something I could no longer escape. I prayed and prayed for God to show up like Superman and start fixing my problems - saving me from my depression - saving me from myself. My prayers seemed to be ignored. *"How long O Lord? Will you forget me forever? How long will you hide your face from me? How long must I wrestle with my thoughts? And everyday have sorrow in my heart?" (Psalm 13:1-2)*

Well, God did not show up in a Superman cape and fix my life. Everyday I felt more and more on the edge. I decided to take a good hard look at my problems. I believed if I helped myself maybe, God would start to help me. The first step I took was to look for a new job. I found a new job teaching English and Math at a learning center. It did not pay as much as my other job and had no benefits program, but I had to get out of the negative atmosphere of my old job. I also realized less money would cause more stress for Randal, which in turn would cause me more stress as well. I honestly no longer cared. I gave my two-weeks notice at the care home and have not once regretted my decision.

Although I changed one area of my life, my other problems still existed, as did my depression and anxiety. I continued to pray for change - change that never came. I thought surely God knows how many problems I have and have no one else to turn to. I was getting very close to the end of my rope. I sat down one afternoon and read my bible. While thumbing through the pages I found a verse I had highlighted years prior. I was surprised to find something so fitting to my present situation. *"Consider it pure joy my Brothers, whenever you face trials of many kinds because the testing of your faith develops perseverance. Perseverance must finish its work, so that you may be mature and complete, not lacking anything." (James1:24)*

I found little comfort in that passage, and I still had all my problems and a deepening of my depression. I failed to see how my upside down life could be viewed as "pure joy". My depression sank to a dangerous level. I had serious thoughts of killing myself. As each day passed, my thoughts of suicide became more and more real. I decided I would wait until Christmas was over before doing it. I knew when, where and how I was going to end this unbearable misery. Events unfolded and my family found out what I was planning on doing. I felt deeply embarrassed and ashamed of myself. I still feel what I put my children through is unforgivable. Of course, they forgave me, but I have yet to do so. I have promised my family that is something they never have to worry about. That dark time is gone forever! It was the love of my children that saved my life and I thank God they did.

Christmas was fast approaching and Lydia was flying up to spend it with us. I still felt very depressed, and I thought it neccessary to get some anti depressants from my doctor. I felt like I had nothing to offer anyone. Randal was very supportive and we were able to begin honest communication about our issues. Our marriage started to improve and we began to show each other respect again. Both of us were relieved we could start mending our marriage and began to work as a team once again. I believed my life was beginning to improve and I was getting excited about Lydia's visit for Christmas.

One evening before Christmas while at work I noticed a pain in my left breast. It was a sickly ache and it came out of nowhere. This pain would come and go, and I shrugged it off as nothing. The pain continued coming and going for the entire evening, and the next day I still experienced this pain. It would come and go as before. The ache was not going away and I told Randal about it. He felt about my breast and told me he could feel a lump. He pointed my fingers in the right spot and sure enough I too felt a lump. It was a hard lump, not very small and situated behind the nipple. Randal took me to the doctor that day and of course the doctor felt the lump as well. He scheduled me for a mammogram and an ultra sound for the beginning of January. I had two weeks to wait for my tests and hoped and prayed it would be nothing serious, but somehow I knew it would be.

Despite my aching breast we enjoyed our Christmas. Lydia stayed with us for one week and I really enjoyed her visit. I had told her about the lump and ache in my breast and she too hoped it would be nothing serious. Randal and the kids as well as my mom worried about the lump. At times I became very afraid, but at times I was sure it would not be cancer. I do not understand why, but breast cancer was something I was convinced would never happen to me. Breast cancer happens to other people, but to everyone else I am other people. I thought I could get cancer, just not breast cancer. None the less I knew something was seriously wrong. All I could do was to pray my same old prayer for God to do something.

Diagnosis Day

Be still and know that I am God. (Psalm 46:10)

WOW! And did God ever do something. "I've seen the results of all your tests and what we have here is cancer. Only cancer looks like that." My surgeon spoke bluntly as I sat across from him stunned and speechless after he had performed a biopsy. By the time I made it into the surgeon's office I had a pretty good idea what he was going to tell me, but to hear it and know it as my reality was shocking. By this time I knew I had breast cancer, but I wanted it to be some kind of mistake - some sort of lab mix up. As I sat there I almost said, "You're kidding me, right?" It was a surreal experience beginning the moment I reached the hospital.

My appointment was for 10:00 AM. I was unable to drive myself to the hospital that morning because the day before I was in a motor vehicle accident two blocks away from home. The day of my accident I had gone to work early to prepare all my teaching plans, as well as my boss's teaching plans. It was January and the roads were very icy. On the way home I hit a rut in the ice, which caused me to go careening out of control and straight into the oncoming lane. The oncoming lane contained a large white truck and I knew I was going to crash straight into it, and I did. My little car was badly damaged, but there was no damage to the big white truck. Luckily no one was hurt, but the only problem was that I no longer had a vehicle.

Randal was unable to drive me to the hospital the morning of my biopsy, because his company had a big job for him to do and it could not be cancelled. My son Matthew was the only one that was able to take me to the hospital for my appointment. When Matthew dropped me off I told him I would phone him when I was finished. Nervously I walked into the hospital and checked into admitting. The clerk that served me called a nurse to escort me to the surgeon's office where my biopsy would be performed. From admitting, I followed the nurse through a labyrinth of doors, corners and corridors, "Very unusual for such a small hospital." I thought to myself. As we walked my mind raced. I struggled to control my thoughts and fears. I was able to control myself. As we were approaching the "destination of horror" I thought to myself, "I have breast cancer. Why else would I need to see a surgeon for a biopsy?" *"O Lord, hear my prayer. Listen to my cry for mercy; in your faithfulness and righteousness come to my relief." (Psalm 143:1-2)*

As I continued to follow the nurse I thought about the day I had my mammogram and ultra sound. I was nervous that day too. As I entered the Mammography Department I had been greeted by a rather large and gregarious technician. She was a lovely lady and really put me at ease. As she showed me the change room she quietly requested, "Strip down to your waist." Those were words I would hear often during the coming months. I did as she instructed and entered the mammogram room with the intimidating machine that was going to squish my breasts. I stood there in the flimsy gown feeling awkward and insecure, wishing it was all over. I looked at the mammogram machine and thought, "There it is, the machine that is going to cause me great pain." I had been told by so many women how painful this procedure is. I stood looking at this machine, calmed myself down and braced myself for this horrific painful experience. The technician asked me if this was my yearly check up. I explained about the lump. She tried to be positive, and agreed when I stated it was most likely a cyst.

The moment I was dreading arrived. It was time to place my left breast on this machine. I was nervous as the procedure began. The technician made all the proper adjustments and then my breast was getting squashed. I was amazed by the lack of pain. I had anticipated a pain that would be almost unbearable, but it was just somewhat uncomfortable. She repeated the same procedure on the right breast. She directed me to the waiting room while she checked the photos to ensure I did not have to repeat the procedure. As I waited I wondered what the outcome of the mammogram will be, "What if I have cancer?" "What will happen to me?" "If I do have cancer, will it be terminal, or will there be hope for me?" I could not imagine having a serious illness and wondered how it would affect my life and my family. The technician returned to the waiting room and she pleasantly escorted me to the ultra sound room. Still wearing the flimsy gown I sat down and briefly waited for this next procedure.

Once on the bed, I was asked to open my gown. I was bare breasted as the ultra sound technician put the cold gel on me and began the exam. This lady was very different from the one that performed the mammogram. This technician was very, very quiet. She did not speak a word to me and was very methodical in her work. She pressed down on the area where the lump was and as she did so it stung. This was far more painful than the mammogram and it seemed to go on for hours. She concentrated her exam on the same area, the lump. Her lack of conversation made me very nervous and I though, "Oh, I definitely have cancer." I knew she was measuring the lump. I wanted so desperately to be someone else, but I was me and I was getting these tests because I have cancer - "Oh God, help me please!" When the ultra sound was over the quiet technician politely told me I could get dressed and leave.

As I continued to follow the nurse to the surgeon's office my nerves became worse. I knew a serious storm was blowing into my life, and I had to get to shelter as quickly as possible before my life was lost forever. "I am a cancer patient now, God!" My prayers became more and more urgent on this seemingly endless journey to the surgeon's office. I begged God, "No matter what, please let me live long enough to watch my children grow and marry. Jesus, please let me live long enough to hold at least one grandchild." I then thought about my mother, "Jesus please let me die after my mom. Oh God, it would break her heart to bury me - her only daughter." I begged God for my life as Jesus once did, *"Abba, Father," He said, "everything is possible for you. Take this cup from me. Yet not what I will, but what you will." (Mark 14:36)* I fought back the tears as I prayed to God for the strength to be able to get through this labyrinth without breaking down. I needed strength to hold back the floodgates until I was alone.

Finally we arrived at the surgeon's office and he was there to escort me to his examination room where he would perform a biopsy. Once in the examination room I once again was told, "Strip down to your waist and put this on." Another flimsy gown. I nervously did so, and awkwardly climbed up on the exam table. I looked around the room. Odd thoughts one has under great stress. I noticed he had beautiful dark wooden cabinets, and I thought, "Those are very expensive cabinets." As I lay waiting for him to enter the room I wished it was all over. He walked in and asked me to undo the gown and sit up. "Oh God, how humiliating," I thought. "A man I just met seconds ago is going to look at my bare breasts while gravity allows them to sag!" I did as he asked and he looked at my breasts at eye level - closely! Could this get anymore embarrassing? My eyes wandered nervously around the room while I continued to wish this could be all over. "You never noticed any changes in your breast at all?" He asked. "No, nothing." I replied as he shook his head in disappointment. He then asked me to lie down in order to perform the biopsy. I stared up at the ceiling while he took a firm hold of the lump and reached for some sort of medical tool. Soon the procedure was completed and it was time to get dressed. When I sat up to dress myself I noticed the biopsy sitting on the cabinet. It looked gross. It was a brownish greyish color and I thought, "That doesn't look healthy."

I came out of the examination room and sat down across from the surgeon at his desk. Before he spoke he was doing some paperwork, and I took this time to look around his office. I studied all his neatly framed medical credentials and took stock of all the items on his desk. I looked at him and wondered what his life was like. He was a tall handsome man and I believed by his wedding band he was most likely happily married. I wondered what his wife looked like and if she worked. I thought she was probably a happy woman enjoying the perks of being a surgeon's wife. I wondered how many children he had and how old they were. Then he spoke.

I listened in stunned disbelief as he continued, "Your tumour is quite large. It is about 2.5 cm. You will require a full mastectomy." "Oh my God, I'm going to lose a breast!" I thought to myself. He continued some more, "I believe that is your best option. I could give you a lumpectomy if you wish, but I feel that would be inadequate." "Oh my God, I'm going to lose a breast!" I thought again. "If I give you a lumpectomy you will only be left with ¼ of your breast and you could also be at a greater risk of recurrence." "Oh my God, I'm going to lose a breast!" That was all I could think about. I had thought if I had breast cancer, all I would need would be a lumpectomy. To hear otherwise only added to my shock. "Do you have any questions?" At that point a few tears escaped from the prison I had forced them to remain in. I took a tissue from the box on his desk that I had noticed moments earlier and wiped my eyes. I just sat there in shock, not really believing what I had just heard, while at the same time knowing that was exactly what I was going to hear. A few more tears rolled down my cheeks and he patiently waited for me to respond. As the warm salty tears rolled down my cheeks uncontrollably, I gathered up enough strength to ask, "Will I be able to have reconstruction?" I've never had much breast pride, or thought they were beautiful, but at least I had two!

The thought of losing a breast terrified me and saddened me deeply. The surgeon reassured me reconstruction would be an option for me. I could not believe I was having this conversation. The only breast surgery I ever would have considered was an augmentation, but it was never a priority in my life. Now breast surgery was my number one priority and hopefully would help to save my life. It truly is amazing how quickly a person's life can change. He finished our appointment with the usual doctor speak, "Your surgery will be very soon and the hospital will contact you when they have a date." It came time for me to leave and as I was walking towards the door he said, "I'm sorry I have to give you this news today." I replied with a shaky, "Thank you." He gently patted me on the back before I walked out the door.

So, there it was. It was official. I had breast cancer. I was a true bona fide cancer patient. The surgeon's words rang through my head as I traveled back through the labyrinth of corners and corridors. I walked into the hospital that morning thinking I might have cancer and now I was leaving the hospital knowing I had cancer. I was full of fear and uncertainty more than ever. I felt so insecure and afraid walking through the hospital. I looked at people and envied them. I believed I was the sickest person in the entire building that day. My prayers had become more desperate than before. All I wanted to do was go home. I found the pay phone and called Matthew to come and pick me up. I waited at the main entrance of the hospital for him and all I could think about was, "I have cancer." I dreaded having to tell my loved ones.

Matthew was the first to know. I watched him pull up in his truck and I immediately ran out the door and into the safety of his vehicle. He looked at me and I looked at him and I began to cry as I blurted out, "I have breast cancer!" I can't even remember our conversation. I was in so much shock, but I know I repeated everything the surgeon told me, and I remember he was upset. We drove home and once there I told him he had to go and get Grandma. I phoned Randal after Matthew left, and I relayed all the gory details to him. His words revealed his shock and I could hear the shock in his voice. He was sorry he could not be with me and I wished so much he could. I felt alone and scared. I had to phone my mom next because Matthew was already on his way to get her.

This was the phone call I dreaded the most. How does a daughter tell her mother she has cancer? I gathered up my courage and dialled her number. My heart sank when I heard her say, "Hello." I broke the news to her and I clearly remember what she said, "Oh Wendy, no!" I then told her I had to have a full mastectomy and again she said, "Oh Wendy, no!" I told her Matthew was on his way to pick her up and I kept our phone call very brief. I told her we would talk when she got to my home. When I hung up the phone I cried. I cried because it broke my heart to tell my mom her daughter has cancer.

While I waited for Matthew and Mom to arrive I phoned my other mother Lydia. I bravely broke the news to her. She said almost the exact same thing as my mom, "Oh no Wendy!" She told me she had a feeling it was cancer, but hoped she would be wrong. I could hear the disappointment and concern in her voice. Both of us wished we lived closer, so she could be with me. I also told her about my car accident the previous day and she felt terrible about that as well. Neither of us could believe how much bad luck I had in just two days. I cried when our conversation ended.

Just as I hung up the phone Matthew and Mom walked in the back door. The oddest thing happened. Suddenly my feeling of total fear was gone. Truly gone! I felt strong and calm. I had to be strong for others, especially my mom. We decided to order a nice lunch in. Matthew phoned Nick and he came to have lunch with us. While we waited for our lunch to arrive our visit was interrupted by a phone call.

It was a close family friend, Jean. Lydia had phoned her and told her the bad news. Jean had breast cancer 15 years prior, and has been cancer free since. As soon as I heard her voice I began to cry and exclaimed, "Oh Jean, I don't know what to do!" "You're going to do everything your doctors tell you to do." Jean's words were able to calm me down and I found comfort in them. She gave me much advice, sympathy and empathy. She told me she had a wig a friend of hers had given her and she would put it in the mail the next day. I was excited about that and anxious to get it. I was able to stop crying and we ended our conversation with, "I love you." When I got off the phone with Jean I felt much better and I felt relieved I knew someone that had already been through what I was about to experience.

After I hung up the phone my mom walked into the kitchen to ask me what Jean had to say. That was when I saw tears in my mom's eyes and the last thing I wanted was to see my mom cry. I always felt heartbroken whenever I witnessed my mom cry. I walked towards her and calmly said, "Oh Mom don't cry. This is going to be okay." I gave her a much needed hug. She held up very well that day and I was glad she was with me because I really needed my mom that day.

Nick arrived at the same time our lunch showed up. Nick, Matt, Mom and I all sat down at the dining room table and ate our lunch together. God really does work in mysterious ways, because this meal seemed like a celebration. Honestly, from that moment I felt a strong sense of adventure. "Am I crazy?" I wondered to myself. Maybe I felt a sense of adventure because I had been in such a depressive rut for so long that anything new or different seemed like an adventure. Personally, I believe it was the work of God. He gave me what I needed to accept the shock and be strong for others as well as myself. We really enjoyed our impromptu lunch.

The only member of the family that still did not know about my cancer was Melissa, another person I dreaded having to tell. Matthew picked her up from school and I told her when she got home. Everyone including Melissa knew about my lump and tests, but she too hoped it would be nothing. Obviously, she was as upset as everyone else. Nick and Mom came over after he finished work and all of us, but Randall spent the evening together. I enjoyed having the kids and Mom around me. We were a real comfort for each other and I thank God I had them with me.

Night crept its way into the day - my diagnosis day. All my phone calls were made to important family members and friends. Mom and Nick had returned to their homes, Matt and Melissa to their rooms to do their teenager things. I sat alone waiting for my husband to come home. I grew more and more impatient for Randal's return home. While sitting alone waiting I began to think about my uncertain future and reflect on my recent past.

Again, amazing how fast life can change. Now I was a cancer patient. My perspective on life now changed forever. I had thought life was something hard that happened day after day. I remembered how angry I used to be every morning when I woke up. I also remembered how just a few weeks ago I wanted to end my own life. How selfish - how utterly selfish I was! How cruel that would have been to do to my husband, my children, my mom, close family members, and close friends that truly cared about me. What a terrible legacy I would have placed upon my children, my children for whom I would do anything. I had believed I was alone in this world. I even thought God gave up on me, that he quit listening to me like a parent exhausted by its young child's relentless and immature demands. I stopped believing in the promise Christ made, ***"...And surely I am with you always, to the very end of the age." (Matthew 28:20)*** Now, while alone

I felt God's peace and knew he was listening when I prayed. Although I did not know if I was going to live or die I knew he was going to save me. I also realized in addition to listening to me he was also with me when I was broken hearted, ***"The Lord is close to the broken hearted." (Psalm 34:18)*** I felt the shame of a sinner that evening. I cried, "I have cancer and I want to live! Oh God, please forgive me for even thinking about ending my life - my life you created! Oh Jesus, I'm so sorry! I'm so very sorry for what sorrow I caused my family to feel!" Cancer is perfect, absolutely perfect at putting everything into proper perspective.

Randal arrived home close to midnight. He hugged me and did all the husbandly things husbands do at such a time. We spoke about my day. He wanted to hear all the details. He asked me questions I could not answer; something that would happen frequently in the coming weeks. He wanted to know if I planned on working until my surgery. I explained that I had just been hit by a tidal wave of shock and going to work and dealing with children was the last thing I felt I could do. He seemed disappointed, but I didn't care. Money comes and goes and this was my time. It was all about me now. The past three years had been all about depression, anxiety, heartbreak, loneliness, neglect, rejection, work, and enormous stress. Now it's about me and healing me, ***"A time to kill, and a time to heal. A time to breakdown, and a time to build up. A time to weep, and a time to laugh." (Ecclesiastes 3:3-4)***

Randal went to bed before me that night and once again I felt alone. Everybody was asleep. I cried, oh how I cried. I cried because Randal wasn't with me on the worst day of my life. I cried because I had been so selfish and foolish weeks before. I cried because I did not want to say goodbye to my children. I cried because I may not live long enough to watch their lives develop. I cried because I missed my dad. I cried because I knew how sad my mom felt. I cried because I was scared. I cried because my body betrayed me. I cried because I had to lose a breast, and I cried because I wanted to cry. I stayed awake all night. I prayed most of the night, "Oh Jesus help me! Oh God will you stay with me all night because I need you. Will you listen to your daughter? I am so sorry for everything I have done wrong. Please God stay with me all night. Oh God, please help me." As the hours ticked by, God and I continued to be together as Father and daughter.

Diagnosis day was over. I was diagnosed with breast cancer on January 28, 2008.

Waiting for Doomsday

Peace I leave with you. My Peace I give you. (John 14:27)

My first day of knowing I have breast cancer was now behind me. Because I was awake all night I witnessed everyone wake up and leave for the day. Again I thought about my cancer. I did not think about it in a depressing manner. I thought about it in a curious manner, "What will happen to me? When will I have the surgery? What will it be like to have one breast? How will I look with only one breast? How will this effect my marriage? Why did this have to happen to me? Why wouldn't it happen to me? How did I get cancer? What did I do to cause this?" Oddly I was no longer depressed. For the first time in years I had a positive attitude. Of course I still had feelings of fear, anxiety, and uncertainty; that is only to be expected. That morning I was anxious to have my mastectomy. I knew once my left breast was gone my cancer would be gone. I just couldn't wait to have this thing taken off of me.

After everyone was gone from the house I went up to my bed and caught a little sleep. I only slept a few hours, but when I woke up I was genuinely happy to get out of my bed and live a new day. Odd as it may sound, I had something to live for now. With my new positive attitude I felt strong. Gone were my feelings of despair, hopelessness, and desperation. I was given the gift of inner strength and peace. God gave me a positive attitude, while releasing me from the heaviness of my depression. The beauty of this gift is that He gave it to me freely. I did not ask for this gift.

He gave it to me freely and I finally had the peace I so desperately needed before, now and in the coming months. God finally answered my prayer.

A positive attitude is essential when battling cancer. I believe it is just as important as the medical treatment. I was fully prepared to fight this battle tooth and nail with all my might. I had more than enough arsenal. I had a positive attitude, a fighting spirit, medical treatment and God. I was in the fight for my life. I compared it to the Old Testament story of David and Goliath. David felt empowered after conquering the lion and was confident he could conquer Goliath. I was like David and with God's power I felt confident I could conquer cancer - Bring it on! *"You come against me with sword and spear and javelin, but I come against you in the name of the Lord Almighty…This day the Lord will hand you over to me; and I'll strike you down and cut off your head." (Samuel 17:45-46)*

The thought of losing my breast was difficult for me to accept. Before the surgeon told me it was coming off I assumed all I would need would be a lumpectomy. I was heartbroken about it. Everyone is different and I had no intention of taking a chance on a lumpectomy. Better to lose a breast than my life. For most of my life I have had a love/hate relationship with my breasts. I loved having them for obvious reasons, but was never satisfied with their size and shape. I was a 36 C, but would have preferred to be a 36 D! Breasts are so important in society today and I was going to have only one.

Older women have expressed to me the female breast has always been exploited within society. Yes, I agree whole heartedly, but I believe this exploitation has escalated over the years and it has become a complete obsession. One just needs to look at the plastic surgery industry. Breast augmentation is the number one cosmetic procedure for the western woman. It is no longer for the rich and famous. For many years the rich and famous fuelled this industry, but now plastic surgery is something many people choose to have. One thing I find disappointing is many young women and young girls tend to base their worthiness on their breast size. This is pathetically sad given the fact women have so much more to offer the world than their breasts.

For me the importance of reconstruction is to gain back what I lost. I want to be even again. I fully admit I hate, absolutely hate walking around this world with just one breast. Everyday I resent having to put on my mastectomy bra. I have lost some self-esteem, and I realize having reconstruction is not my only means of correcting this - but it will help. I encourage any woman of any age to have their breasts reconstructed if it is important to them. For others that do not want to have reconstruction that is their perfect choice.

I named the day of my mastectomy, "Doomsday", because that is how it made me feel. While waiting for Doomsday I had to see my family doctor, Dr. Thomson. He had a positive attitude and believed with treatment my chances were good. I had a list of questions for him to answer, but he couldn't tell me anything about what my treatment would be. I wanted to know what to expect. Will I have to have Chemo? Radiation? He told me an oncologist will give me a treatment plan and that won't happen until after I recover from my mastectomy. That is just the way the system works. He assured me that all my questions would be answered at the appropriate time. I must admit I left his office disappointed. I just had to be patient and I knew being patient would be difficult for me.

My frustration worsened when family members would ask me the same questions I was asking. It was as though people thought, because I had breast cancer I had gained a wealth of knowledge about it overnight. I did some research about it on the computer, but found most of the information general. When others asked me questions all I could say with honesty was, "I don't know." I explained to everyone that I would see an oncologist after I had healed from my surgery. That led to the next question, "How long after you heal will you have to wait to see one?" Again I would respond, "I don't know." "Where will you go to see one? Do they have an oncologist in Fort St. John?" "I don't know." My personal favourite, "What's an oncologist?" My family and I were not stupid. We never had to deal with this before - simply put; we were inexperienced. Regarding my father's cancer he had seen an oncologist quickly after his diagnosis, but his cancer, was terminal. He was told he had about nine months left to live. He died after three months.

During this period of time I felt somewhat abandoned by the medical profession. "You've got breast cancer. Your tumour is too big for a lumpectomy, so we're going to cut off your breast. Sometime in the future, can't say when, but you will see an oncologist. Can't tell you what your treatment will be. You might have to have chemotherapy, radiation - don't know yet. Okay then, they'll phone you with an appointment sometime in the future...Phone if you have any questions." I have spoken to other survivors and they have admitted they had the same experience. I was just left to hang in limbo. Limbo came to an end - sort of. I was scheduled at the hospital for a pre-operative examination and scheduled to meet with a nurse. I have had nine surgeries, so I knew exactly what to expect. The pre-operative examination went as usual. I was much more interested in meeting the nurse. I hoped maybe she would be able to answer some of my questions.

I was reading one of those gossip rags when the nurse called me into her office. I walked in, sat down and became instantly nervous. I was surprised by how young she was. She was an attractive young lady with a bubbly personality, and she quickly put me at ease. She was so eager to help and so anxious to please. She asked me if I wanted to go and meet the chemo nurses. She expected me to get up and follow her to meet them right then and there. In retrospect, that would have been the logical course of action. I would have had some of my questions answered, but I had suddenly become weird. I declined. She then suggested booking me an appointment for that very day to have a bra fitting at a specialised shop. I declined. She asked me if I had any questions and I said, "No." She slumped back into her chair seemingly defeated by her inability to help me, or please me. Knowing she was disappointed I felt frustrated with myself. I refused help. Maybe I was not yet ready for what was being offered. I also knew I came off as aloof and I felt I hurt her on a professional level. I had to explain myself, "I'm not trying to be difficult. I'm just stunned. I'm not ready for any of this today. I'm just stunned." She smiled and said she understood. She gave me her card, invited me to phone her when I felt ready, and before leaving she gave me a "cancer kit".

This cancer kit was great. It was a white case and had plenty of literature in it. It contained a book all about breast cancer written by leading Canadian specialists. The kit also contained numerous pamphlets and booklets all related to breast cancer. It was a complete A-Z about breast cancer. There was a small booklet written by the Canadian Cancer Society with pertinent phone numbers. There was also a booklet about the mastectomy, chemotherapy, radiation, hormones etc. etc. I was so happy to receive this case and the pretty young nurse smiled at me knowing she finally did something to help me.

When I arrived home I checked my mail and I was unexpectedly excited. Jean's parcel arrived! I was thrilled and quickly ran into the house and opened my parcel like an excited little girl on Christmas morning. There it was - my first wig. I put it on and was blown away! It looked exactly like my own hair. It was the same color and style. I kept looking in the mirror feeling so happy - something new, and something positive. Jean also included a pink ribbon and a coin with a pink ribbon in the middle of it.

While wearing my new wig I made myself a cup of tea and I sat down to read all my new literature.

Later Melissa came home from school with her boyfriend. Still wearing my wig I waited for them to say something about my hair. I was surprised when neither one said anything at all about it. I waited a little longer and still not a word from them. Finally I said, "Don't you notice anything different about me?" They both looked me up and down with puzzled looks on their faces. They admitted they could not see anything different about my appearance. Suddenly I pulled the wig off my head and watched their jaws drop. We shared a good laugh. Shortly after Matt came home with one of his friends and I repeated the same scenario. After Matt picked his jaw up from the ground he said, "I just thought you backcombed your hair a little more." I played that trick on everyone and no one once suspected I was actually wearing a wig.

That was the most eventful experience I had while waiting for my surgery date. I spent most of my time waiting, reading, watching T.V., playing computer games, visiting with my mom and I went out for coffee with my friend, Joanna. I also spoke to another good friend of mine, Juanita over the phone. Randal and I spent most of our evenings together talking and watching a few of our favourite T.V. shows.

As each day passed without hearing from the hospital I grew more and more anxious and frustrated. I phoned the hospital 4-5 times hoping they would give me a date. The last phone call I made the nurse at administration became cranky, so I decided not to phone anymore. One Sunday afternoon Randal and I were just hanging around the house together when the phone rang. Finally!! Finally they gave me my surgery date - Tuesday morning. The nurse instructed me to shower the night before, not to eat anything after midnight, remove all my jewellery, and to be at the hospital by 6:30 am.

After hanging up the phone, my positive attitude and sense of adventure suddenly vanished. I became overwhelmed with sadness. It hit me like a ton of bricks - my days of having two breasts were almost over. I relayed all the information to Randal. The day of my diagnosis he told his employer he would not be at work the day of my surgery - and this Sunday he phoned and confirmed it. I was relieved Randal was going to be with me throughout the entire day. Randal was being very optimistic and quickly noticed my entire attitude had changed. He asked me why I had become so quiet and withdrawn and then I began to cry. I could not talk I was so upset. He tried to comfort me by saying, "You know I am going to be with you through everything." I appreciated that, then blurted out, "It's not that!" How do you explain to a man how profoundly sad it is to lose a breast? I didn't know how to explain to him why I was crying so hard. He sat in silence not knowing what to say or do. I cried for several more minutes. I wished I was someone else. I wished God would change my situation.

I knew God wasn't going to suddenly heal my breast, but I didn't know how else to handle the sense of doom hanging over my head. After a few more minutes of crying I somehow found the strength to tell Randal, "I don't want to lose my breast. I want to keep it and be healthy. I want to have two breasts! I don't want to go to the hospital and become disfigured. I am so sad this is happening to me!" I still can not put into words how sad and alone I felt. There was nothing Randal could say or do to take away my fear and sadness, and I didn't expect him to. It was what it was and I had to face it bravely. I knew I had my family and friends behind me, and I knew God was still in control of everything. Randal did say something to help me feel better about my future disfigurement, "You're still going to be you." The rest of the evening was very quiet.

The night before the surgery I followed the nurse's instructions with both relief and resentment. I felt relief to have the cancer removed and resentful I was in this situation. Randal and I went to bed and the both of us just laid there. I guess he was dealing with what he was feeling and I was doing the same. I was completely withdrawn and talking about it was not going to help. Randal understood I had to be within myself. I don't think either one of us slept a wink - I know I didn't. I watched each hour pass by on the clock. I turned off the alarm at 5:29 am before the horrible buzzing sound could annoy me. I think the worst sound in the world is the sound of an alarm clock. I wondered why I even set the stupid alarm knowing I wouldn't sleep all night. We both quietly got up. There wasn't much to do before leaving for the hospital. I could not eat or drink anything. There was no need to style my hair and I couldn't wear any make up. All I had to do was get dressed. Randal showered and had his breakfast, and for the first time in our marriage I had to wait for him to get ready. While waiting I contemplated the events of the coming day. I was so sad! It came time to leave and I didn't want to go. We left.

The hospital is only a 10 minute drive from our house. On the way I sat quietly, not uttering a word. All I felt was great sadness and all I could do was pray for strength to get me through this upcoming nightmare. We arrived on time at the hospital and we went through the usual check in procedure. Oh, how I resented everything! Another very pretty young nurse escorted us to a room with a bed. I envied her remembering when I was her age and didn't have cancer. She showed me the lovely attire I was to change into and handed Randal a large bag to place my clothes in. Pleasantly she told us she would be back in a few minutes.

I removed my boots, pulled down my pants, took off my tunic, took off my sweater, reluctantly removed my panties and socks, and with great sadness removed my bra. I thought to myself, "I'll never wear that bra again." With great resentment I put on the flimsy green gown, pulled up the funky long green socks and placed upon my head the ugly green cap while Randal packed up my clothes in the bag. We didn't speak a word. Once I finished putting on the entire hospital garb I laid down on the bed with my legs slightly crossed and my arms resting on my chest with my fingers interlocking. I then laid there and stared up at the ceiling.

The nurse returned and when she saw me lying there as I was she began laughing. I began to laugh as did Randal and I jokingly stated, "I'm ready to die." A little comic relief was much needed to break the tension. The nurse hooked me up to the I.V., gave me a sedative, told me to go for my final pee at 7:15 and informed me the surgical nurses would come and get me at 7:30. I prayed God would give me what I needed, as I no longer knew what I needed anymore. I looked over at Randal sitting in the chair beside me and he looked very forlorn. I felt sorry for him. I quietly said, "I wish this didn't happen." He quietly replied back, "No shit." He took me to the bathroom on schedule for my final pee and we went back to the bed to wait some more. We sat in silence again - and then came the nurses. It was time to go. I looked at Randal and I saw the concern in his eyes. His face revealed he had his own inner turmoil. He told me he loved me and reminded me he would be there when I woke up. Oh God, why?

Away I went. I was so scared, my butterflies had butterflies. They steered me through the hallways until we reached the operating room. Before wheeling me in there (that dreaded room), they asked me what my name was, when I was born and what procedure was I having. I got all the questions right and they said it would just be a little longer. I lay in the bed in front of the operating room feeling like the whole world went on a wonderful vacation and forgot to take me with them. I felt alone and afraid. I felt even more alone and afraid when a nurse came and said, "Okay, Wendy here we go."

Once in the operating room everyone introduced themselves and explained their roles to me. They were all in good moods and at times tried to get a giggle or two out of me. If I remember correctly I giggled once. I was glad to know the people I was putting my trust in were happy, but I still felt afraid. I can remember wishing this was happening to someone else. I then thought, "This is happening to someone else somewhere else in the world." I then wished I was one of the nurses, heck I wished I could be anyone else, but me. I prayed, "God be gracious and let me wake up from this when it's all over." Everything appeared to be ready, but there was one key element missing - the surgeon.

The medical team started asking each other about the whereabouts of the surgeon. No one knew where he was and he should have been there by now. One of the nurses went to find him, and returned minutes later to explained why he was not there yet. I almost gasped out loud. The nurse spoke pleasantly, "It seems the surgeon has slept in this morning. He is finishing his morning coffee and will be here soon. I guess he is allowed to be late like anybody else." I nodded my head and said, "Yes", but I thought, "Oh God, he slept in? Are you kidding me? The day I'm having a mastectomy he sleeps in! Please God don't let this be a bad omen." The anaesthetist took mercy on me and put me out before the surgeon arrived.

Just before I was put out I gave my breast one last thought. From the day I was diagnosed, January 28, 2008 until this day, February 11, 2008 I did not once look or touch my left breast, nor did I say goodbye to it. I didn't always appreciate it, but I really did love it as much as every other part of my body. I knew how greatly I was going to miss it. Only now as I write do I have the strength to forgive my body for betraying me and the strength and peace to say goodbye. Goodbye left breast and thank you for all your years of service.

Doomsday

Weeping may remain for a night, but rejoicing comes in the morning. (Psalm 30:5)

Today as I sat down to write this chapter I couldn't shake the depression that cancer patients often carry. Earlier this week I had to go to a hospital in Grand Prairie, Alberta to have a central line put in my body. I really wanted this, so I would not have to be poked all the time anymore. While in Alberta we were able to shop for my daughter's birthday before going to the hopital. After the fun en route to the hospital I took two Lorazepam as I was really nervous. The thought of having a tube inserted into a vein in my arm and threading it through until it sat above my heart gave me the creeps. The procedure was supposed to take about one hour, but because my veins are deep and difficult to find it took almost two hours. Due to the Lorazepam I was able to relax and even doze off a few times. When it was all done I was wiped out, and relieved it was over.

Today I had to have my bandages changed and site cleaned. I wasn't feeling well emotionally and physically, but I had health obligations I could not ignore. I walked into the chemotherapy room and the nurse was caring for two other ladies. Usually this wouldn't bother me, but today it depressed me. One lady was quite elderly. I could see her I.V. and in addition to clear liquids she was receiving a blood product. The other lady was about 70ish and she was completely bald the way I used to be. There was nothing unusual about them or what was being done to them. It was just me.

Before the nurse attended to me she had to care for both of them first. I sat in one of the recliners and discreetly watched. That was when I began to get depressed. I wondered to myself, "Is this chemo room nothing but a holding tank for those who will soon die?" Nothing seemed positive to me. I felt so low. I was feeling depressed that I was still going through chemotherapy. I thought about what my life was like before I got sick and felt melancholy. I wished my treatment was over. Some ladies I met in the chemo room were a little ahead of me and now they are done. Their chemotherapy and radiation is long finished. They are on hormone treatment and two of them are even back to work, but here I sit in the chemo room. I was so jealous!

The nurse was able to attend to my bandage and clean the site. She explained everything she had to do as I carefully listened. It only took her 15 minutes and then she was free to attend to the others again. My hair was coming back, but I still had to wear a wig. I started to put my wig back on and I was thinking about going to the doctor after this to get more medications. Always getting more medications. I get so sick of it! The thought of driving around the block to my doctor's office on this cold December afternoon made me want to cry. It was such a cold northern day. At least there was no wind chill. I continued to put on all my winter gear and with a sigh I ventured out into the cold again.

I arrived at the doctor's office (and because they know me so well due to my weekly visits), the receptionist had my file and was waiting for me before I even had my boots off. I was surprised when I looked up and saw her waiting for me. We shared a quick little giggle and then she led me to one of the examination rooms where I waited for Dr. Thomson. Not much of a wait. Dr. Thomson walked in with his usual positive manner and smile, and sporting a suntan. He had just come back from a 12 day vacation in Costa Rica. I told him how much I miss him when he takes time off, and how one gets very accustomed to one's own doctor. He laughed and I complimented him on his tan. I wondered if I would ever have the opportunity to have such a wonderful vacation. Oh well, my life is what it is now and I have to concentrate on getting well. He wrote out the usual prescriptions and made an order for me to have more bloodwork done. I started to dread going back out into the winter before I even left the room.

I got myself back into my truck and dreaded going to the pharmacy. I just wanted to be in the warmth of my own home. When I arrived at the pharmacy they were very busy and I was so fatigued. I was disappointed when they told me I would have to wait one half hour. I had to pick Randal up from work at 5:00pm, so I decided I would pick up my prescriptions then. Back out to the cold outdoors to get home for a couple of hours and try to warm up. I took some Oxycodone to help relieve the body aches. My aches didn't seem to want to go away today. I had waited patiently for them to go away, but they persisted. I spent my few hours in Randal's recliner wrapped up in a wool blanket in an attempt to cure me from the chills I had caught from outside. I waited patiently for the aches to go away, but the pain was still there. I prayed God would let these pills do their job and that He would help me with my depression. My time had run out, and I had 15 minutes left. I started the truck so it would be warm, and invested another 10 minutes in the recliner.

I got up, put on my long hair wig, my toque, my matching scarf and winter coat. I put on my boots, grabbed my purse, opened the door, faced the cold air and with determination shivered my way to the truck. I went to the pharmacy to pick up my meds, some groceries, and then pick Randal up from work. By the time I arrived at the store I noticed my body pain was considerably eased and my chills were gone. Walking in the parking lot to the store I thanked God for small mercies and was able to accomplish all my errands. It always surprises me. Just when I think my emotions are under control something - even something small happens and puts me in a cloud of despair. It does pass though. That is the hope one has when battling bouts of despair and depression - it does pass. Now this odd day is done and I can relax and rewrite chapter four.

The first thing I can remember after waking up from my surgery was a nurse at my bedside. I do not remember what she was doing, but I noticed my self medicating Demerol drip beside me and gave myself a couple clicks. I noticed Randal was not in the room, but more importantly I remembered why I was there. I felt my left side where my breast should be and it was completely flat. My cancerous breast was gone, *"He cuts off every branch in me that bears no fruit." (John 15:1)* I thought to myself, "It's gone, it's really gone. Forever gone." I couldn't think about anything else. Tears began to slowly roll down my cheeks, and I turned over onto my right side and quietly cried myself back to sleep.

Later, somewhere between sleep and consciousness I could hear a nurse speaking to Randal. She was angry with him because he clicked my Demerol drip for me. She was firmly telling him he is not to do that - it is for me to do, and she explained he could give me an overdose. I thought what Randal did was thoughtful, not wrong. He knew me well enough to know that I would appreciate the gesture. I felt bad he was being scolded by a nurse and thought she was making a big to-do about nothing. Those self-medicating drips are set, so there is no chance of an overdose. Again I drifted back to sleep.

The next time I woke up I was more alert and saw Randal sitting in a chair at my bedside looking at me. I said to him, "Where have you been all day?" He giggled and replied, "Right here, you've been out of it all day." I was doubtful, so I stated, "but I woke up and you weren't there?' He explained the only time he was not there was when he went for lunch. I knew he was there for me even if all I did was sleep. He asked me if I remembered him and a nurse lifting me from one bed to the one I was now in. I had absolutely no memory of this. Randal was surprised because he had asked me to lift my butt, so that they they could get me in the bed. I apparently said, "Okay.", and lifted my butt just like I was asked to do.

Randal and I were enjoying our conversation when a good looking nurse walked in and said, "Hi Wendy." I replied back with a polite, "Hello." I assumed she came in to take my temperature and blood pressure, so I resumed my conversation with Randal. She remained standing and I wondered what she wanted. She said, "Wendy, I'm Leah" During a short pause I thought, "Am I supposed to know this person?" She broke the awkward pause with, "Leah, Krystal's mom." Suddenly it all became clear to Randal and I who this woman was. She was Matt's friend's mother. Matt and Krystal had made Leah promise to come and see me when she was working. I felt terrible knowing how horrible I looked, but I couldn't do much about it. Now that we knew who and what was going on we had a pleasant visit. We talked about our kids of course, but we also got to know each other better. She was a very nice lady and was a truly a bright spot during my hospital stay.

After Leah left I started to loose steam. It was about 3:00 pm and I told Randal he should go home and get some rest. He took my advice and I quickly fell back to sleep. When I woke up Randal was back, and I told him I had a headache and was feeling nausea. I always get a migraine and nausea when I have surgery, because of the anaesthesia. As we sat together and talked my supper tray arrived. Due to my nausea I gave my supper to Randal. I noticed my headache was getting worse, and I knew it was evolving into a migraine. The nurse gave me something for it and my nausea. By the time Randal finished his supper I started to drift off to sleep again. I could hear Randal talking to the nurse about my milk. He asked her to put my milk on ice because, "She loves her milk cold. The colder the better. When she wakes up she will have cold milk to drink." I was blown away by that! How thoughtful. When I heard Randal instruct the nurse about my milk I thought, "That's what love sounds like." What a beautiful moment in my marriage! I did wake up a little later and thanks to my husband I enjoyed my cold milk.

Randal came back to the hospital in the evening. When I woke up again I was surprised to see him at my bedside watching me. He looked so exhausted. He had no sleep the previous night and spent almost the entire day beside me. We talked a little, but I could tell he was having a difficult time due to his exhaustion. He mentioned he talked to the surgeon who told Randal he was pleased the surgery went well. He believed all the breast tissue was removed. Randal continued talking, but I interrupted him telling him to go home. It was about 8:00 pm and I would only be going back to sleep. I told him I didn't need him to stay and he needed to get some sleep. He was reluctant, but I did convince him to go home.

I woke up frequently during the night. I would stay awake about a half hour. I could feel the headache getting worse as well as the nausea. I looked at the shadows on the walls. It reminded me of the times I was in the hospital having my babies. Those were special times in my life. Each baby offered such a unique experience. My favourite time was when the nurse would bring me my baby during the night for feeding. Once my baby was satisfied I gazed at it and enjoyed the purity of the love between us. I completely delighted in their presence. It was a wonderful and peaceful time. It was the calm before the storm. Soon the nurse would return and take my newborn back to the nursery. I would lie there and watch the ways the shadows rested on the walls while thinking about my baby. It was a quiet comfort and always made me feel warm and secure. This time in the hospital with my mastectomy I watched the shadows on the walls and didn't derive any comfort from them at all. The shadows made me feel sad and lonely and I wondered if life would ever be good again. ***"You will grieve, but your grief will turn to joy." (John 16:20)*** Let's hope so!

During the night the nurses would make their rounds. They would come in and take my blood pressure and temperature, and I found it very annoying. I knew they had to do their job and it was for my own good, but I couldn't wait for them to leave. I tried so hard to go back to sleep, so I didn't have to once again lie there thinking about the reason I was in the hospital. Between the nurses, headache and nausea it was impossible to sleep well. I could only sleep between two to three hours and then wake up again. It was a terrible night, and a lonely one.

The next morning the surgeon came in early to see me. He asked me how I was feeling and I told him I had a migraine, and about my worsening nausea. He ordered medications for both. He asked me if I looked at my left side when the nurse changed the bandage. I told him I did not, and he said to me, "You are going to have to look at it sometime." I politely agreed, but inside I felt furious. Did he think he was telling me something I didn't already know? Did he think that I was going to get through the rest of my life without looking at it? Did he think he knew how I felt? I suppressed my anger. He informed me I would be spending another night in the hospital. I didn't care; in fact I was relieved to stay another night. I knew it would be best for my health to remain in the hospital one more night. It also gave me more time to be alone with God. That gave me comfort.

Early that morning my close friend Juanita came to visit me. Her husband had some early morning tests at the hospital, so she spent her time waiting for him with me. It was good to see her. We worked at the same care home together and became close friends. I truly love my friend Juanita! While we were visiting I told her about my migraine and nausea. The medications the doctor ordered had not yet come my way and the Demerol would only work for a little while. The nausea would come in waves. Juanita and I were only able to visit for a short period of time. Juanita was talking to me and I could feel the nausea getting worse. I knew vomiting was imminent. I looked at Juanita and told her straight she had to leave because I was going to be sick. I was polite about it and she understood perfectly.

Shortly after Juanita left Randal walked in. He wanted to see how I was doing before going to work. I told him about the migraine and the nausea, and how they were getting worse. Not much Randal could do about it, but I didn't expect him to. He still looked exhausted and I told him so. He admitted he didn't sleep at all the previous night, because he couldn't stop worrying. I asked him what he worried about, and I clearly remember his words, "About you and what it's going to be like. If you'll always be sick like this." I told him we would just have to wait and see. I suggested he stay home from work and get some sleep. He declined stating, "We need the money." As long as I've been with Randal we've always needed the money. We had a serious illness in our family, but we were in it together. We just had to deal with all the upcoming situations together and take things as they come. I knew Randal was going to be by my side throughout the coming months and I felt more secure about our marriage.

The rest of my morning was a battle on two fronts - migraine and vomiting. The doctor and nurses were doing all they could to rid me of these two ailments. I would click my Demerol drip a few times and my migraine would ease. Then I would get a wave of nausea and vomit, washing away the relief the Demerol gave me. This pattern continued the entire day.

Matt and Melissa came to visit me on their lunch hour, bringing me a bag of chocolates and a bouquet of flowers. Melissa always cries when she goes to a hospital. When Randal was in the hospital with pneumonia the previous year Melissa came with me one evening to visit him. As we were leaving I looked at her and noticed her crying. She asked me if Randal was going to die. I explained Randal's health issue and reassured her he would be coming home in a few days. This day I looked at her and I could see she was forcing herself not to cry. During their visit the nausea hit again and they soon left. Matt came again after school with his friend. Not five minutes into the visit and I started to vomit again. Randal came to check on me after work. He was just in time for my supper to arrive, and he enjoyed it again. Mom and Nick came in the evening, and didn't stay long due to my vomiting. Randal came back in the evening and helped me when the nausea waves hit me. He left when visiting hours were over. I wished him well and hoped he would have a good night's sleep. I hoped I would have a good sleep as well. My migraine was now a nagging headache, but the nausea was still an issue. Again I looked to the shadows on the walls for comfort and again they failed to comfort me. My second night was just as lonely and sad as the first.

I thought about my left breast at great length this night. Having one breast is so unnatural to me and has deeply affected my sense of being a woman. It has also caused me to fear my sexual relationship with my husband. Randal is a breast man. His attraction to the female breast has always made me think about Proverbs 5:9 regarding my breasts, *"...and may you rejoice in the wife of your youth. A loving doe, a graceful deer- may her breasts satisfy you always, may you ever be captivated by her love."* Oh God, here I am married to a man that loves breasts and I can't even give him two anymore. Yes, this is going to be a nagging concern for me for some time.

When morning came I still had a headache and nausea. I slowly made myself get out of bed and pushed my I.V. into the bathroom. I saw myself in the mirror and what a fright! Leah was working again and stopped in to see me. I felt so embarrassed knowing how horrible I looked, but we had a pleasant visit. We talked about my mastectomy, and it was comforting to have a woman to talk to about it. She shared her health issue with me and we both felt better knowing we understood how each other felt. I enjoyed Leah's visit for 20 minutes without once being interrupted by vomiting. I was getting better. After Leah left a nurse came to show me how to drain and measure the liquid from my drainage cup, which I found terribly GROSS. That was when I first saw my left side. My mastectomy looked like all the pictures in my books. My left breast had been replaced by one long red line. I wasn't as upset as I thought I would be, but I did feel some anger and resentment. I drained the cup well and was very confident I would be capable of doing this easily.

Shortly after a familiar nurse came in and gave me something different for my headache and nausea. After about a half hour those terrible side effects from the anasthesia were finally gone. Randal arrived at the hospital to help me get dressed and take me home. I didn't really want Randal to see my chest, but he wanted to. While getting dressed I allowed him to look. All he said was, "cool." I thought it was an odd choice of words, and assumed he chose that word so as not to make me feel worse about it. What else could he say? "Wow, that looks really gross." or " That looks really good."

After Randal helped dress me we gathered up all my belongings and left for home. I could hardly wait to get home and on my couch. It is always so true - there really is no place like home, and I love my home. Randal had all my favourite foods for me. My mom came to visit and the three of us just sat around and talked. Everybody felt better once I was home. Now I just had to recover from surgery.

It was a slow process, but I was lucky because I had no complications. During the first week I had numerous phone calls from concerned family members and friends. My close friends came to visit me bearing either chocolates or flowers. As time passed I healed. One of my best days was when my drainage cup was removed. I felt very good at the end of eight weeks and was looking forward to the next step.

Complete and Utter Turmoil

Commit to the Lord whatever you do, and your plans will succeed.
(Proverbs 16:3)

The course of cancer treatment offers patients a wide array of experiences including delays, successes, new friends, support, disappointment, enlightenment, emotions, the list goes on. One experience that often comes about is the unexpected. As I was beginning to write "This is my Cancer" the unexpected paid me a visit. I was forced to stop writing chapter five and go through this exhausting and unexpected period of time. The unexpected put me in a very depressive state followed by great inner joy.

When I finished my second round of chemotherapy I was feeling great. It was October and feeling healthy I decided to start walking daily. The weather was wonderful and all us northeners were enjoying our fine weather before the snow and cold arrived. My mom and I enjoyed walking together. I was feeling so healthy and energised I applied for a part time job at Walmart. I wanted to make some extra money for Christmas, and I was happy and almost certain the future was going to get brighter and brighter.

My oncologist phoned me in October. She had wanted me to fly down in August for a check up, but I was too sick to travel. When she phoned me this time making the same request I was feeling good enough to make the trip down to Vancouver. I invited Matt to come along as he needed a holiday and he loves Vancouver. Matt came with me to all my appointments and was able to spent some time with one of his close friends living in the heart of Vancouver. I spent the remaining time at my brother's house in Mission. They were away on holidays in Arizona, so I had quality time to spend on my book and enjoy visiting with my nephew and his family who lived in the basement apartment. It was a really good trip.

Upon my return home I was still feeling healthy. My knees were sore, but I thought it was nothing serious. It was now nearing the end of October and mom and I were still enjoying our daily walks. Everything was clipping along nicely, but in a matter of two days everything changed. Certain events occurred, shook my world and forced me in a state of confusion, frustration, and turmoil - complete and utter turmoil. Suddenly everything in my life seemed unbearable. Nobody around me could understand what I was going through. I felt I was losing control as each event piled on top of the other.

The first event was not serious, but I was very disappointed. While in Vancouver I phoned Walmart to enquire about the job I had applied for. They told me they would let me know about my position the next week. The next week came and no phone call, so I phoned them, "We are still processing your file." Blah, blah, blah! I felt put off and disappointed. I wanted this job so much. I could make extra money for Christmas and bring some normalcy back into my life.

Next my oncologist phoned me and informed me my MUGA scan showed my heartbeat had slowed down due to the Herceptin treatment. She explained Herceptin is known to do this, but it wasn't serious. My treatment was going to be delayed by one month in order for my heart to to regain a normal heartbeat. I was so disappointed about this because the last thing I wanted was a month's delay, prolonging my treatment.

Next my family had issues to deal with. Issues with children and husbands do not disappear just because one is undergoing cancer treatment. These issues are very personal. I felt like screaming at my family. I reminded myself they had been supporting me for months, and it's not easy to watch their wife and/or mother be sick for months. They had their own issues, fears, and setbacks to deal with. I had to remind myself these issues were in no way a personal attack against me! I cried for many nights without letting anyone know how stressed out I really was.

The major family issue that shocked my world was the day I was told Matthew was gay. I already knew he was gay when he was a very young child. I cannot explain how or why I knew, but my motherly instinct told me "This boy is gay." I believed for many years I would be well prepared for the big day I got the news. No such luck. I took it very hard. Maybe it was not being told he is gay, but how I was told.

One dull evening Melissa was doing her laundry when I went to talk to her. She looked me in the eye as she was gathering up her clothes and stated, "Matt's gay" I thought she was angry at him about something and was kidding around. I giggled and shrugged it off. She continued doing her laundry and once again looked me in the eye and stated very seriously, "No Mom, Matt is gay." "Oh this must be some kind of joke." I so hoped this was a joke. "No, Mom Matt is gay. He told me." I immediately began to cry, "This can't be true." "Mom it's true. It's okay. I cried too when I found out." Oh God, my son is gay!! Do you hear me God? My son is GAY! GAY! This is not the life I would have wanted for him. All those suspicions I had all his life are true. My son is really and truly gay. This is reality. This is my reality. I have never had issues with the gay community and always believed they should have the same rights as the rest of the world, but my son is gay. My first question was, "Are you sure he is gay, maybe he is bisexual?" I hoped so desperately Melissa would tell me, "Yes Mom, he is bisexual and tends to desire women a little more than men." Oh no, instead, "Yes mom, he is sure." My next question was, "Why didn't he tell me this when we were together in Vancouver?" Her answer broke my heart, "He didn't have the guts." My son was too afraid to tell me he was gay and had no idea I had known this all his life. I cried. I told Randal the big news and he calmly said, "So, he's still Matthew." "Yes, but he's gay." Randal tried to be a comfort, but his efforts failed. I then phoned my mom. She agreed with Randal. "But mom, Matthew is gay. He's gay!" I cried for most of the night. The next morning I had to take my mom to see Dr. Thomson and I secretly hoped he would be able to do something about this for me, some how, some way.

Mom and I sat in the office waiting for Dr. Thomson the next morning. He entered the office in his usual pleasant mood and attended to my mother's needs. I sat in my chair like a bald lump on a log with a frown on my face . Dr. Thomson couldn't help but notice my utter despair and kindly asked, "Wendy, what is wrong? You look so forlorn sitting there." My mom blurted out for God and everyone to hear, "She just found out her son is gay." Did she have to say it like it doesn't matter? My sweet mother continued, "And he's such a nice boy." Dr. Thomson smiled and said, "They usually are." Oh God, why me? Where is the nearest noose I can go slip my neck into? But, oh the best was yet to come…. I should say a few weeks later I was able to laugh with Dr. Thomson about it. One morning during one of my visits Dr. Thomson started our visit by asking me how my son was to which I replied, "He's still gay." Dr. Thomson said it was good I could laugh about it as he giggled.

Matthew was picking me up that day for lunch and to talk about his big news. I was shocked by how nervous I was to see him. I was shaking and so afraid I would start to cry in front of him. He pulled in the driveway and my stomach sank. Oh God here it goes. I gracefully got in his vehicle, put my seatbelt on and quietly prayed for the strength to speak without crying. I opened the conversation with my usual wit, "How is work today?" I was so nervous I didn't even care to hear his response already knowing what it would be. I nervously waited until we were driving when I had to find out if it was really true, "So, are you bisexual or are you 100 percent gay?" Oh God please let him tell me he is bisexual. His answer was disappointing, "I'm 100 percent gay." Oh God, no - not 100% gay! I so would have settled for 50/50! I managed to make it through the hour free of tears, but when I got home I let go. I made sure Matthew knew I still loved him and supported him just as before. I told him how I had always known he was gay, and it made no difference to me. I didn't let anyone know I cried for two weeks.

The last event was the one that pushed me over the edge. I was coming down with a sinus infection, so I wasn't feeling well. My mom needed me to do her grocery shopping for her. I drove to her house, picked up her list and went to her favourite store. I was unfamiliar with the store, so it took me a while to find everything. I ran into an acquaintance that knew about my cancer. She is a pleasant young lady I taught at the learning center. She proceeded to tell me about her mother. Her mother battled with cancer for seven years. It began with breast cancer and eventually spread to her lungs and brain. She did not survive and she was my age when she died. This really scared me, and once again I became frightened I may not survive. I finished the shopping, dropped off my mom's groceries at her house, then went home and broke down.

I had become extremely angry, and I was trying to identify other emotions I was experiencing. I knew I was slapped in the face by fear. My anger and fear were accompanied by confusion, and the frustration I was experiencing made me all the more angry. My emotions were well over the boiling point and I honestly felt I was about to lose control. I can remember thinking, "Surely, this is what a nervous breakdown feels like. Oh God, what is going to happen?" I had visions of myself being taken away in a straight jacket and living out the rest of my days in a padded cell. It was either that or die the same way that my acquaintance's mother had died. I had to scream - scream out loud exactly everything that my mind had to release. After doing so the writer in me sat down and wrote my exact thoughts. There is some offensive language, so please forgive that and understand. I refuse to edit it.

Ah! Fuck it! Fuck it all! I am going to wallow in self pity and love it. I feel like rolling over and giving up. Why fight? For what? More years of struggling, more years of disappointment, more years of fucken depression weighing me down - down to a pit of lonliness and despair?!

I heard things about a woman that died of cancer. So what makes me think I am going to make it? What makes me think I am going to be cured and live happily ever after? When have I lived happily ever after? Why do some people have so many blessings in their lives? Why do some people have everything while others have nothing?

I'm tired! I'm so tired of breast cancer! I'm tired of walking around one tit less! I'm tired of scars! I'm tired of chemo! I'm tired of side effects! I'm tired of setbacks! I'm tired of depression! I want to roll over and - dare I say it?! Saying it - will that make it happen? Will it come true? I've got to say it! I feel like rolling over and dying! I'm so damn tired of being disappointed! Oh God hear me! I'm so fucken tired of it all!

After screaming and writing out my inner emotions, I was exhausted both physically and mentally. I still felt as though my life was falling apart and I was sick of it. When will I be able to feel secure about my life? As I stood up from my writing table I immediately felt my life was collapsing again. I felt like the devil was standing above me laughing at me in an "I told you He doesn't care about you" manner. I felt so alone and felt my problems were hopelessly unsolvable.

I sat down with my Bible hoping to find something - a word or two - that I could find some comfort in. I came across a verse I have always found interesting. **"Dear friends, do not be surprised at the painful trial you are suffering, as though something strange is happening to you. But rejoice that you participate in the suffering of Christ, so that you may be overjoyed when His glory is revealed. (Peter 4:12-13)** "Okay, that's nice." I thought. Another verse about how wonderful it is to suffer. I decided to have a shower hoping at least my body might be calmed.

I love a hot shower, so I had the water perfectly adjusted and allowed the water to soothe and calm my body. I focused on prayer as the water rained upon me, and I prayed relentlessly for peace. With nobody home I was able to pray out loud. Over and over I prayed for peace. My experience with prayer is that there is a significant period of time before God answers a prayer, but this day was different. I was in the shower for at least one half hour and as I was thinking it was time to get out, I suddenly felt God's presence very strongly. It felt like He was reaffirming with me to keep going and that I was doing what I was supposed to be doing. Peace came over me. The peace I had prayed for half an hour ago was upon me and it energized me. My body was still somewhat restless, but I allowed the water to continue to rain on me before stepping out.

Reluctantly and slowly, I came out of the shower, dried myself off, wrapped my body in a towel, and climbed the staircase to my bedroom to dress. I was still alone in the house. I could feel God's presence. It was as though He was very close, slightly above me. I looked towards that direction and felt afraid. I was afraid of His greatness and I began to cry. With strong conviction I thanked Him for His peace, His presence and His encouragement. As I wept, I promised I would do what He had asked me to do. My emotions grew deeper and deeper and I felt His greatness - truly felt it! I wanted Him to stay, so I kept praising Him. I continued to praise and thank him, and I felt such joy - joy I cannot explain. At one point I didn't know if I should laugh or cry, so I did both. I fell to my knees and yelled out to Him:

As you have directed me to do, I will do - for your glory - for your name! Thank you for giving me this task. I am honoured you have asked me to serve you. Oh God, Oh Father, Oh Jesus You are real! I can feel you!

Praying, thanking, praising, laughing and crying all before my Lord. What a day!!

I must pause here and admit I had heard of this "joy", and this "peace", and this "glory" before and never understood it, doubting it was true. When I heard others' testimonies and they spoke of the joy, peace, and being in His glory, I found it difficult to believe. Maybe because I had never experienced it. When I became a Christian at 16 I felt I was in God's presence, but never felt anything like it since. I also had strong doubts when others would speak of being close to God - intimately close to God. My level of closeness to God has come to be like this. I am now at a deep level of my relationship, believing - and joy. Now I can be open to so much more in my faith and my walk with the Lord. Despite my illness I now have that "joy". Thank you God!

Slowly I began to become calm and was able to rest, realizing how powerful God is, and how His children are not strong enough to see him in His full glory. This experience was not short and I knew enough time had gone by that someone may be home. They would have heard me. This worried me because I didn't want anyone in my family to think I was upstairs going crazy. I quickly went downstairs to ensure I was still alone in the house. Luckily no one had come home. I felt so wonderful inside. It was a beautiful feeling knowing Jesus had been so close to me and comforted me as I had been so desperate for it. I went back upstairs and felt strongly compelled to write. Although I had become calm I still felt some level of elevation. I could feel the adreneline rushing through my body as I sat down to write. The words came without thought. My hand wrote the words, but God is the author! The following is what transpired.

Want cancer? Be negative.
Want life? Be joyful under the Lord.

Accept death as it is real - here
Accept life as it is and has always been
Real - Believe and you shall see.

No more negative thoughts, actions, words,
live life in abundant joy as God gives it
freely.

Why does God allow suffering?
Because it leads to life.
It leads to Him.

When He calls you to serve, will you hear?
Allow room for the ridiculous 'cause
it will lead you to pure joy!

Feel your pain and consider your pain
felt by everyone in the world in every age,
and that is what Jesus felt upon His cross.
His blood atones for all sin.

God is joyful when His
child comes to Him. Just
like a parent is joyful when
their child comes to them.

Place your eyes upon the
finish line. Place your deeds
upon the finish line,
because the finish line
is where it really starts!

Rest in Him when suffering
as He comforts His children
as each child needs it
- uniquely.

The Lord has breathed
life into you, exhale
and share your life.
Give it to Him with
much thanks. And love
Him, with every breath
He gives you throughout
your entire life.

Recognize the lies of the devil
and let them fall at your feet.
Stomp on them until they no
longer have power, then on
your knees, thank you Father.

Accept each other as we are.
When this is not done we
are rejecting God's handiwork.

God made us as we are.
He will never condem us
for how He handcrafted us.
He made us perfect - allow
His perfection to bring joy
inside you and your house.

Have you loved an insect?
If so, you will love that

same insect again.
Have you loved an animal?
God keeps that animal for
you to love again.
Have you loved a human?
That human waits for your love again.
Have you loved yourself
Why wait? Love yourself.
Have you love for your Father?
Your Father has love for you.
He waits for your love -
Let Him in and all will make sense.

How true - Death is Life!
Find comfort, this wonderous
mysterious foretelling is true
Do not panic - Let Him
comfort you, show you - it will happen.

There is a place!
There is a place God has made
for His children that believe
in him and love Him.

We are a work of art
created by the Father - Our Father
is an artist. What artist paints
the same picture over and over?

We stand as dirty rags before
His greatness, but blood cleans us
up in order to serve and
to serve Him is divine calling.

Rejoice and cry out for
Thanksgiving, once you see
the hand of God work
within your life.

Let yourself find the signs
He has put out for you. For
His signs are truth and
leads to Greatness within
Your soul.

His blood atones for all sin.
Do not insult Him when
regarding other people's sins.
Nobody's sins are better or less
sinful than anybody else's.

Sin is Sin
Death is Death
Life is Life,
and God is God.
Do not try to change Him
to suit your needs, wants,
or desires.

Shine your light bright as
Jesus so desires you to do so.
Jesus shines His light upon
You, so you will shine your
Light for others to see.
As seeing is believing.

See through your soul
because that is where
you will find him.

Love your brother and sister!
When you do, you love yourself
and this gives God His Fatherly
pleasure.

To rebuke Christ is to deny life.
To rebuke Christ's brothers and sisters
is to rebuke Christ Himself.

To rebuke God's son is like hating
your brothers and sisters, breaking your
Parents' hearts and breaking God's heart.

God looks upon you daily,
minute by minute.
What do you want Him to see?

Everyone knows within their
soul, deep within their soul
that their Father is real.
One only needs to accept it
and then life will truly begin!

A parent loves their child
no matter what - So God
loves you. Be humble and
let Him love you - that is
the perfection of this world.

Every great work by
every great artist
has flaws we do not see.
So we have flaws
God sees, but still we
are a great piece of work!

We are as we have been made.
We grow as we have been destined.
We are destined as we have
been called.
The calling is always present
answer the call and find joy,
as that is where it dwells.

The human heart is strong
enough to love everyone.
When in doubt of this, ask
Jesus to show you.

The human heart is weak
enough to hate everyone.
When in doubt of this,
ask Jesus for strength as
hate is the beginning of hell.

We do not know the ways of
God. We do not know the mind of
God. We do not know what God
has for us, but it is good because
God is good.

Heaviness of the heart weighs
us down. We do not see
who keeps us up. All we
know is we are still standing.
How - Who - The Father!
The human heart will physically
ache when broken hearted.
The divine power of God will
console it! Allow this relief,
as it strengthens the soul.

After this experience I had become physically and mentally exhausted. I had already been suffering from a sinus infection, and the infection became considerably worse. I became quite sick for two weeks, and was unable to write about this experience. I was angry about being too sick to write . Now that I am well I am able to give this chapter special attention. I do not know what purpose He has for these little verses. I do not claim anything. I was inspired to write these verses, and if anyone finds comfort in them that is beautiful. Look at them as poems written for you by a breast cancer survivor.

Reassurance

"Because he loves me." says the Lord, "I will rescue him;
I will protect him, for he acknowledges
my name. He will call upon me, and I will answer him;
I will be with him in trouble, I will deliver him and honour
him. With long life I will satisfy him and show him my salvation"
(Psalm 91:14-16)

I felt much better having my surgery behind me. Although my breast was gone, so also was the cancerous tumour that invaded my body. My physical recovery from the mastectomy did take as long as predicted. I was back to my normal physical self by the eighth week. In the first two or three weeks I had sharp shooting pains caused by angry nerves. These pains really hurt, but they were fleeting. The drainage cup was bothersome. It was always in the way and I strongly disliked draining it and measuring the liquid. It made having a shower a real pain. I couldn't wait until that thing was gone. I had no complications and honestly nothing to complain about.

I spent a lot of my time lying on the couch watching T.V. I soon grew bored with that, especially during the day. I tried to take up a couple of hobbies, but soon lost interest. My close friends came to visit me and took me out a couple of times. During this time I read all the literature I had been given. I was able to confirm what the doctors told me about my cancer. I knew I had stage two breast cancer and realized I was a hair's length from stage three. I read all about the treatments and the side effects of those. I assumed my next course of treatment would be chemotherapy.

As I slowly regained my strength I grew very bored and had to look for something to do. Some days I found something to do and some days I found nothing. Randal and the kids carried on with their usual activities. This period of time was uneventful for me - the calm before the storm, or should I say - storms. I grew more and more impatient with the hospital in Vancouver. They were to phone me with appointments to see an oncologist, radiologist, and a series of tests. I had phoned numerous times, but they never had anything to tell me. Weeks passed and still no contact from them. Even a survivor friend of mine thought this was a long wait. Two months had passed and still no word. I felt this was an unreasonable amount of time to wait. Randal told me that if it were him he would phone and demand some action, and yes - Randal would do that. With Randal's inspiration I made another phone call. With a certain tone the woman on the phone said, "Once we have all your information we will contact you." I was angry by this woman's attitude. I felt like shouting, "I'm worried sick about my health. I am a cancer patient. How would you feel if it was your life?! Hurry up and do your job!" I kept my cool. I decided not to phone again. I just had to wait and think - and think.

I couldn't help but think about dying. That is perfectly normal and to be expected. I have always had a fear of dying. At times in my life this would be very crippling. A major component of anxiety is the preoccupation with death. At times this preoccupation would become very bad; very difficult for me to manage. I told a Christian friend about my fear of dying, hoping she would offer some comforting and encouraging words. No, she just said, "It is wrong for a Christian to be afraid to die. If you truly believed in God you would not be afraid." "Gee thanks," I thought. Of course this made me feel guilty, but I reasoned it out. I was a true Christian and a fear of death is part of human nature and as already mentioned a part of anxiety. I believe the notion that true Christians do not fear death is an unfair assumption. Just because a person accepts Jesus as their personal saviour doesn't mean they no longer experience fear. A fear of death is part of human nature and it is neither right or wrong. I was never afraid of where I was going after death, but I was afraid of how I was going to get there after my last breath. The following analogy is how I explain my fear of dying. I call it "Fear of Flying".

Unexpectedly I win a trip to Hawaii. I have always wanted to go there. I know it is a real place, and all the pictures I've seen of it show it to be a paradise. I'm so excited and can't wait to go. There is only one problem. In order for me to get to Hawaii I have to fly and I have a fear of flying. I know I have to go, but how am I going to get through that flight?

One night during my recovery I was prevented from falling asleep due to my fear of death. I was so scared that my death would be soon and I felt heartbroken I would have to leave my family - that I would have to say "Goodbye." As much as it pained me to think about leaving the ones I love and missing out on so much of their lives, this night was spent fearing death more than anything else. I remained downstairs in the living room while everyone else slept. I did not bargain with God - I merely begged for exactly what I wanted in return for nothing. I prayed, " Please God, don't let me die, please give me more time. Please don't let me die now. Please, all I want is more time. Please let me live long enough to see my children grow and marry. Oh God, please don't take me yet. I'm so scared! God I'm more than scared, I'm terrified! Please let me live long enough to hold at least one grandchild. Please don't let me die before my mother. I don't want my mom to experience the hearbreak of losing a child." I told God how deeply I believed in Him and I told Him I know where I am going after I die. I used to say "I believe in God/Jesus/Heaven because I have to." - meaning I believed all that "God stuff" was true, but never actually felt the reality of it. I had to believe it, especially in hard times.

My breast cancer was definitely "hard times" and of course I believed because I had to. Now God was about to show me a better way to believe. That night God gave me a "sense" of the dying process. It is difficult to explain how God released me from my fear of dying, but I am determined to explain it. I was looking out the living room window at the winter's night sky and told God about my fear and suddenly a sense came over me. I sensed very strongly that dying is nothing to be feared. A second sense came over me that Heaven is a real and physical world. Accompanying this sense was a sense of size. I sensed Heaven as a real physical world that is beyond anything humans can fathom. The only way I can describe this is that it reaches out beyond the entire universe. Consider the size of humans and the infinity of the universe, and try to comprehend it all. Although we are no bigger than a grain of sand we will live in a physical world that has no end. Our God is everlasting, Heaven is everlasting, God's children will live with Him in everlasting life. Hard to bend the mind around a world that has no borders, no time, abundant joy, abundant and pure love for everyone and for each other! We will be a family and He will live among us. A third sense came upon me as I looked up at the stars. I sensed (as well as imagined) when I die, as I walk away from this world, everything about this world will fall away from me, from my being. The beauties of Heaven will begin to be part of my being (a part of my new reality), as I approach this new world. Finally God put inside me the "feeling" of reality of the written word regarding Heaven. When Heaven is mentioned in the Bible I can feel its reality. I did not see into Heaven and do not know what it's like, *"No eye has seen, no ear has heard, no mind has conceived what God has prepared for those who love Him." (1 Corinthians 2:9)* All I can say with absolute certainty is it's exactly as described in the scriptures. All this sensing and feeling was incredible. I felt so relieved. Gone, gone forever is my fear of dying. I'm not afraid of flying anymore. That was one of the greatest and glorious gifts God has blessed me with and I'll never forget it. Praise God, He comforts and teaches His children well!

Although my fear of dying was completely gone, my fear of dying at this point in my life still scared me. As I praised God for releasing me from my fear of death I continued to pray God would give me more time. For the rest of the night I begged God for more time. It was early morning when I stopped praying and went upstairs and quietly crawled into bed. I was careful not to wake Randal as he had to get up in a couple of hours and go to work. He was still snoring as I settled myself comfortably in our bed, and I began to pray again that God would give me more time. I prayed myself to sleep.

I woke up around 10:00 AM. My cancer and dying were the first things I thought about. Randal and the kids were gone to work and school. My emotions were mixed. I was still feeling the effects of God's wonderful and much needed gift. I was so grateful God cured me of my fear and so excited how marvellously He worked within my life. I also felt heartbroken that death was a real possibility and saying "goodbye" was something I couldn't even bear to think about. I lay in bed and thought about everyone I knew that has died, especially my dad. What a day that was.

It had been a Sunday when I drove to my parent's house to visit Dad. He was very very sick. He was no longer my dad. He was a different man - he was a dying man. He had withdrawn himself from all of his family, and the process was upon him. Before going into his bedroom to see him, my brother Terry took me into the living room and told me his death would occur very soon. The public health nurse had just left the house and left behind for us a paper with a list of symptoms of approaching death. Terry told me he had many of them. I began to cry. He gave me a brotherly pep talk, told me to dry my eyes and go be with him. I did so. I immediately noticed his eyes. Hard to describe the eyes of a dying person. He looked at me, but his eyes appeared as though he was looking right through me - like I wasn't there. Terry and mom had been up most of the night with him and they were tired. Terry did not want to be there when Dad died. I know this because I know my brother. He said he had to go back to the mainland for his diabetic meds before his pharmacy closes, but before he left the three of us discussed my dad when Mom said, "I don't think he is getting any better." Terry gently told her he would not get any better - that this was it.

After Terry left, my brother Bryan and his wife Delphine came to the house to be with Dad. Bryan and I looked after Dad while Mom got some much needed sleep. As the day progressed it was evident that his death was coming closer. I mentioned this to Bryan and he said, "He could live another two weeks." I thought to myself, "Am I the only one who is not in denial?" I knew my dad would die that day, and so did Delphine. We were all around him when his breathing began to slow down. His breath got slower and slower. Then it got real slow and I knew this was it. I felt a panic jump up into my throat from my stomach and I almost shouted, "No Dad, don't go!" I controlled myself. Bryan and I were on the bed with him. Bryan quietly said, "Go Dad, go sleep with the angels." I remember thinking "What a wonderful and beautiful thing to say." I then told Dad, "It's okay Dad, you can go. We will take care of Mom." I know he heard me as his head turned my way and he looked at me. He then died. Bryan shut dad's eyes for him. After a few moments Mom, Bryan and Delphine left the room. I remained lying beside my dad. I told him everything I felt. I told him he was the greatest man I ever knew. I told him no other man will ever love me the way he did. I told him how much I loved him, how important he was to me and how much I would miss him. I lay beside my dead father for ten or more minutes talking to him and kissing him goodbye. It was the most peaceful day I have ever experienced.

Now I cried while thinking about my dad's death. I still miss him and long to see him again. I continued to think about death and other people. I thought about people that die young. I thought about children dying. How unfortunate for them and their families. I thought about how they had to say goodbye to their families and how hard it must have been. I thought about how hard it would be for me and my family. I also thought I had to get out of bed and get on with the day. I decided to push my fears away and not think about dying.

Later that week Dr. Thomson phoned me one the evening. He phoned to find out how I was and to let me know about the biopsy on my lymph nodes. Four out of thirteen nodes were positive for cancer. Randal and Melissa were sitting there when he phoned. I don't understand why, but at that time I was not bothered by the news and told my husband and daughter in a matter of fact tone. They were quiet and I remember thinking, "I hope I didn't worry them." It wasn't until later I realized just exactly what that news meant.

Once again everybody was in bed and I was still awake downstairs watching T.V. I wasn't even thinking about my lymph nodes. I picked up my breast cancer book and read about the different stages of breast cancer again. I realized the magnitude of having cancer in the lymph nodes. I realized the magnitude of my illness, and it hit me like a hurricane! This is bad! Once again I became terrified I was going to die, and again I was heartbroken at the possibility of saying "goodbye" to the ones I love so much. "Please God, let me live longer. I don't want to die yet." I was facing my own mortality and that is so very terrifying. No one can know how that feels until they themselves are in the same situation. Now I knew how other people that have a serious life threatening illness feel. TERRIFIED! This was another night I spent begging God for more time. "God please, please, please just give me more time." I must have cried an ocean that night as I prayed so hard for God's mercy. I went to bed about 5 am and again I prayed myself to sleep.

The next morning I woke up early and waited for everyone to leave the house before I got out of bed. I felt absolute dread. I depressingly trod downstairs, and spent the most part of the morning crying. I was so disappointed about the results of the biopsy. I was also disappointed because even though God had released me from my fear of death I was suddenly still very much afraid I was going to die. I could die soon! I could die soon! Now with the realization of the seriousness of my illness, my soul had become heavier. I prayed for hours. Was there anything else I could do?

Matthew had come home unexpectedly from school that morning. I didn't have time to wash away my raccoon eyes left over from crying and Matthew instantly noticed. He knew immediately something was wrong - very wrong. He insisted that I tell him. "Mom, what's wrong?" I could hear the alarm in his voice and I knew there was no escaping telling him about my lymph nodes. It broke my heart to tell him. Matthew demanded, "Mom, what does this mean?" He spoke with urgency and real fear. It broke my heart to see the depth of concern and fear on his face. He kept repeating, "But Mom, what does this mean?" We both knew what the lymph nodes are and we both understood their function in the body. I couldn't bring myself to say, "It means there is a good chance some cancer cells have been released into my system." He couldn't bear to hear it either. I tried to reassure him the best I could, but failed miserably to do so. As upset as he was, he left the house to return to school.

Matthew came home from school at his regular hour and had brought pages and pages of success stories about women that have had breast cancer. He first asked me how I was feeling and I told him honestly, "I am afraid." He said he was not scared anymore. His voice no longer had concern and his face no longer wore fear. Instead of going to classes he had gone to the library and researched breast cancer. He sat down beside me and described some of the stories to me. In some cases there were women that had it much worse than me and survived. Matthew had found some hope and his research gave me hope as well. I felt much better. His being so upset made me feel horrible. I didn't know if I was more upset about my lymph nodes or Matthew's state of mind. Nonetheless, thanks to Matthew's research we both felt there was hope for me. Thank you Matthew!

That night I stayed up late again. Although I was feeling more hopeful I was still very much afraid. I prayed the same prayers and I shed more tears. I went to bed in the early morning again, and when I woke up my cancer was the first thing I thought about again. I waited for everyone to leave the house and came downstairs. I felt such sorrow, such a deep sadness in my heart. I made myself a cup of tea and I sat down to drink it in the living room. I felt so lost and didn't know what to do, so I turned on the T.V. without any real thought. I could not believe what I was seeing and hearing. As soon as the T.V. was turned on, instantly there was a young boy about 13 years of age talking. The first words I heard that day from that boy I will never forget, "If I could tell anyone anything with cancer I would tell them that there is life after cancer. You will get through this and live life again." WOW!!! I sat there amazed, completely and utterly amazed! I put my face into my hands and cried. Jesus heard my prayers and gave me comfort first thing that morning. I knew He was speaking to me through that boy. Some people may not see it that way, but I don't care - I do. Jesus wanted to give me peace and hope. He wanted me to know my situation is not hopelesss, and I will have more time. I felt such a great sense of relief and such an appreciation for Jesus. How merciful to give me peace and hope the very first thing in the morning. How wonderful to hear God's words so exact and so soon! Back was my positve attitude. I knew God was going to give me more time - the time I both humbly and desperately prayed for. Thank you God!

Bonus! Within a few days I finally got word from the hospital in Vancouver. All my appointments had been arranged for April. What a relief! Now I was even more anxious to begin the next step in my treatment. My sense of adventure was back!

I looked forward to going to Vancouver for a few reasons. First of course was getting all my tests performed and meeting with the oncologist and learning about my treatment plan - and the consultation with the radiologist. Second reason, I would be able to visit my brother Terry in Mission and visit with my brother Bryan, and with Lydia on Vancouver Island. Final reason, a short trip without Randal and the kids. A nice break on my own. I would only be gone for one week, but I sure needed it.

This is my Cancer

Strengthen the feeble hands,
Steady the knees that give way
Say to those with fearful hearts,
Be strong, do not fear,
Your God will come
He will come with vengeance,
With divine retribution
He will come to save you. (Isaiah 35:3-4)

The morning of my flight to Vancouver finally arrived. I hate flying by myself, so for this reason I had anxiety. The very reason for going also added to my anxiety. Although I was feeling happy about getting my treatment plan, I was also afraid of what it could be. The depression I had suffered from for three years was gone, but the anxiety was still very much present at times. When I am experiencing considerable anxiety I become very withdrawn. I was very withdrawn the morning of my mastectomy and now I was again very withdrawn. I checked my luggage at least three times to make sure I packed everything I needed, and still I worried that I had forgotten something important. Apart from my anxieties I was more than ready to go.

I flew into Vancouver in the late morning and my brother Terry was there waiting for me. I hadn't seen him in a year and a half, and it was good to see him again. He was looking healthy. From the airport we drove straight to the Vancouver General Hospital for my first test - MUGA scan on my heart. We had some time to kill before my test, so we found the hospital cafeteria. Both of us were very pleasantly surprised. What a great place to eat! A wonderful variety of food and a wonderful atmosphere. We had a lot of news to catch up on, and I enjoyed our visit immensely. I felt so fortunate to have such a great brother! He made me feel happy that day and all my anxiety disappeared. Thank you Terry!

After our lunch we made our way to the Nuclear Medicine department. I was a little unnerved knowing I was going to have a nuclear injection, but knew this had to be done. The nurse began with some blood work and then injected me with the radioactive substance. I had to wait for 15 minutes before the radioactive was ready to give a good pictures of my heart. I layed down on the scanning machine, rested my left arm above my head and relaxed. They took pictures for about 20 minutes and I really enjoyed this test. The room was darkened and I felt so relaxed. While laying there I pondered the recent experiences I had with God, and realized how much closer I had become to Him. He heard my prayers all along, and His plan and His will unfolded as intended. I wanted this MUGA to last longer, and was disappointed when the technician lightened the room and told me I was free to go.

It was late in the afternoon when Terry and I drove to his home in Mission. As we travelled through Vancouver's rush hour and the Fraser Valley, we continued with solid conversation. I was anxious to arrive at his home so I could get some rest as my body was tired. After arriving at his home he settled me into my room and we hung out until his wife Debbie came home from work.

It was good to see Debbie again. We enjoyed a pleasant supper, and we were able to catch up. Terry and Debbie suffered a great loss within their family. Their son, my nephew, was killed in a motor vehicle accident a few years ago on Canada Day. Jason was only 28 years old when he died. I was crushed for them - broken hearted for both of them. It was a dark and shocking time and I still can't imagine what it is like for them now. Debbie is a very strong woman and I was pleased she was able to talk about Jason freely and with real strength. Debbie shared her different experiences about the loss of her son and it is a blessing they both have peace. I know they miss their son in a way I have never experienced, but they continue living a healthy life, while enjoying the rest of their family, especially their two grandchildren.

It felt good sharing my experiences about my illness with Debbie. I was able to speak freely and with ease about how important my faith has been, and the role it has played. She couldn't help notice I had a positive attitude and I admitted I had a sense of adventure about my treatment. I told her about the deep depression I suffered from for three years. How absolutely ironic that is. I had been so depressed about everything both big and small, but when faced with a life and death illness, my depression vanishes in a snap being replaced by a positive attitude, fighting spirit and sense of adventure. Maybe I am weird! It was a great evening and then I retired for my next day's appointments.

When I first entered the hospital, I felt overwhelmed. Even walking towards the building intimidated me. I felt so alone within the big city, and all the people around me. As I walked in I felt like everyone except myself knew what to do and where to go. The administration desk was the obvious place to start. I nervously walked up to the desk and said to the woman, "I'm Wendy Clarke and I have an appointment with Dr. Yates." She gave me some papers to fill out and pointed to the adjacent tables where I could do this. When I finished I handed her back the papers and she told me where to go. I took the elevator to the proper floor, and I could not shake the nervous feeling in my stomach. I stepped out of the elevator and found the administration desk. I again announced whom I was and whom I was to see. The woman behind the desk looked at me and asked me where my papers are. I explained I filled out some papers downstairs, but no one gave me any papers to bring here. I perceived the woman was somewhat put off by me as she said coolly, "You need to bring us your papers. You'll have to go back down to Admission and tell them to give you your papers." Back down the elevator and back to Administration, "Hi, they said upstairs that I am to bring some papers with me." This woman appeared to be in a better mood, but did not know anything about my papers. She asked her co-worker and they both looked around, but saw nothing. They had to phone my doctor's office upstairs to find out what I needed. When she got off the phone, she told me my papers were sent up to the doctor's office the previous day and they should have them.

My nervousness turned to annoyance. Back upstairs where my papers apparently were. Nope. The same woman was there, and she was on the phone. I patiently waited for her to finish and politely told her. "They said downstairs my papers were sent up here yesterday." She looked at me annoyed and looked around her work area and said, "We do not have your papers; they know that downstairs." I thought to myself, "How many times do they do this? Surely they must know what they are doing." Back downstairs I went and told the woman, "They say the papers are down here with you." The woman entered a room behind her workstation, and found my papers. She handed them to me and I took them upstairs. When I handed them over to the other woman she said, "You finally got it figured out." I held my tongue.

I was angry and felt so alone in this hospital. This was all so new to me and I wished so much that somebody were with me. I felt uncomfortable being there and wished this did not happen. I looked at all the other patients and thought they are in the same situation as me. How terrible for them and me. I noticed no one was bald. No one was wearing turbans and I could not tell if anyone was wearing a wig. Could all these patients have kept their hair? Maybe I would not lose mine. Oh God how I wished I was not there alone. As the woman looked at my papers, she told me my appointment with Dr. Yates is at 3:00 pm.

I was more than two hours early. I felt as alone as I did in Japan when I was stranded there by myself. Brief story - while working in Korea my director sent me to Japan to get my working visa. My director sent me to the Korean Consulate in Fukoka on a Korean national holiday - their equivalent to Christmas. There I stood in the middle of a major Japanese city all by myself before a closed Korean Consulate. Panic and anxiety set in very quickly. I did not know what to do. My flight back to Korea did not leave until the next day. I decided instead of getting a hotel room I would just sleep at the airport that night, after all, it was an international airport. I frantically tried to phone my husband in Korea with a long distance calling card I bought at the airport. I tried for four hours to get through. Finally, I got an operator on the line and explained my problem. She put me right through to my home in Korea. I told Randal what had happened and how mad I was at my director. I had noticed that during the past four hours there were less and less people in the airport. When I got off the phone a beautiful young worker at the airport came up to me and told me the airport was closing and I had to leave. Well holy @#*&! My anxiety sharply increased. I was able to maintain my composure and told this young woman my problem. She asked to see all the Japanese money my director gave me for the trip. I did not think I had enough left for a room as I foolishly did some shopping at the airport and had a wonderful lunch. She counted my money and told me I had a lot of money left. She phoned a hotel, booked me a room, and escorted me to a waiting taxi. Thank God for her! The second I entered my hotel room I cried and cried. I had felt so alone and afraid. Looking back, I would have done things differently. I made my morning flight back to Korea. When I set my foot on Korean soil, it felt great to be home. That is how I felt at this hospital minus the panic and fear. I noticed the hospital had a library, so I decided to kill some time reading about breast cancer, but it was closed due to lack of volunteers. I really wanted to find a private place to go to and have a good cry. I just hung around the hospital.

I checked in at 3:00 and waited for one hour before I was able to see the oncologist. I sat in the examination room waiting again. It was a typical room, cold and clinical. Dr. Yates finally came in and I was very surprised. Dr. Yates was a woman. She was very friendly and had a great bedside manner. She spoke with an accent I did not recognize. I asked her where she was from, and she told me she was from Israel. I instantly liked her, and she impressed me with her knowledge and confidence.

She began with a description of my cancer. My cancer was poorly differentiated invasive ductal adencarcinoma hormone positve (Her 2). My cancer was an aggressive one with a high risk of recurrance. Terrific! If I had to get cancer of course I would get an aggressive one. Just my luck! Dr. Yates confirmed I had four lymph nodes that were cancerous. Before telling me about my treatment plan, she expressed her concern regarding the size of my lump, lymph nodes and the aggressiveness of the type of cancer. This frightened me. I understood I was still stage two and I concentrated on that instead of freaking out. After all, I had peace about my life.

As I suspected, the next step in my treatment was to be chemotherapy. Dr. Yates carefully explained the details and I thought it all sounded so complicated. Huge words I did not even know existed. I was to have four cycles of Doxorubicin (Adriamyacin) and Cyclophosphamide every two weeks. At the end of that four-cycle plan, I was to have Paclitexel (Taxol) and Trastuzmab (Herceptin) every three weeks for four cycles. At the end of that cycle, I would continue with the Trastuzmab for an additional 13 cycles. Please understand I did not fully comprehend what I was hearing. The lack of comprehension would cause a big shock in the future. The amount of chemotherapy I was to have surprised me. Dr. Yates explained that because of the tumour size, lymph nodes and type of cancer she believed it best to treat me as aggressively as possible. I trusted her opinion and accepted the chemotherapy plan. I did not really have any other choice.

She also explained to me about the side effects. I had no idea as I listened just how horrible those side effects would be. She told me about the nausea, but reassured me there were very effective drugs for this. She told me I would lose my hair as this chemo does cause hair loss. I was also told about fatigue, mouth sores, diarrhea, body pain, chills, fever, flu like symptoms, etc. This all sounded horrific. I hoped I wouldn't get all of them. Although I still felt a sense of adventure and had a positive attitude I was afraid of the side effects. I had every reason to be afraid.

After discussing the chemotherapy, she examined my mastectomy site. She did not say much about it, so it must have been fine. She took this opportunity to discuss radiation with me. She did not go into too much detail as I was to see the radiologist right after I saw her. Before I saw the radiologist, a nurse came in and weighed me. This nurse also explained some more issues and told me I would be back the next day to meet with another nurse to review my treatment plan. I also had to come back and have a chest x-ray, blood work, and and ultrasound on my abdomen. She gave me a folder with an endless amount of literature and most importantly, a copy of my treatment plan. She soon left and I sat feeling overwhelmed while I waited for the radiologist.

It was after 5:00 pm when the radiologist walked in. He confidently introduced himself and sat down in front of me. He was a very handsome man about my age. His first question to me was if I was planning to have breast reconstruction in the future. I told him yes and his reply was, "Not the answer I wanted to hear." I already knew that radiation could affect the effect of reconstruction. He explained everything about radiation and I was to have five weeks of radiation after eight cycles of chemotherapy. I really did not have much faith in radiation, but I did listen closely to everything he had to say. He too wanted to examine my mastectomy site. Oh God, this was the last thing I felt like doing. I was so exhausted I just wanted to get back to my brothers' house and let all the information penetrate. I reluctantly allowed another exam on my site and afterward, I was so anxious to get out of that hospital.

My brother picked me up after all my appointments were over, and we began our drive back to Mission. It was a long drive back during the lower mainland rush hour. I told Terry everything I had learned that day and broke it to him that he would have to drive me again the next day. We arrived back at Terry's and we enjoyed another nice meal courtesy of Debbie. Debbie and I enjoyed another comforting conversation that evening.

The following day I met with a nurse to go over my treatment plan again. This nurse was very thorough. We sat down in a private room as she explained every single word (and I mean every single word) to me. What they lacked in organization the previous day they made up for with excellent care and communication. I can honestly state this hospital has a great medical staff that truly care about their patients.

After my meeting with the nurse, it was time for my chest x-ray, blood work and ultrasound, which were performed in the later part of the afternoon. Again, I experienced some disorganization, but this day I found it very comical. I went to the lab at the appropriate hour to get my blood work done, and the technician was very pleasant. For whatever reason the lab tech and the x-ray department had me scheduled for the same time. Neither the lab nor the x-ray wanted me at this time, so the lab tech asked me to choose. Since I was already at the lab, I chose the lab. I noticed the look on her face. She was not pleased with my decision. I offered to go to x-ray instead. She was quite relieved and made sure it was not an inconvenience to me. I explained I had to do both anyway, so it made no difference to me. She giggled as she phoned X-ray and told them, "She's all yours."

When I arrived at X-ray they were very busy. There were two female technicians and both of them were buzzing around very quickly. The redheaded tech said, "You have to strip down to your panties and put on the gown. You have to have your ultra sound immediately after you're done here. Do you know where to go?" Just as I was about to answer the ultra sound technician walked up to us and said looking at both of us, "This has to be done quickly because I am really busy over there." Both technicians exchanged polite words regarding me, and the topic of time. The ultra sound tech asked me, "Do you know where I am?" Again, just as I was about to answer the redhead spoke, "You go back and I'll show her." He left and the redhead hurried me down the hall, around the corner, down another hall and pointed to the location. She already turned to go back to X-ray before I actually made it to the location. She looked at me and asked, "Do you know?" I did not dare say no. I nodded in agreement knowing I would find my way. She hurried me just as quickly back to x-ray, showed me the change room and reminded me about stripping down.

I felt so hurried and awkward. I think most people feel awkward about stripping down outside of their own home, and combine that with being rushed a sense of being overwhelmed sets in. I did as the redhead instructed me and went into the x-ray room. She proceeded to move and turn me about quickly. She had an abrupt tone, but she was in no way rude. "Okay don't move." I was glad to get out of there when it was finished.

I had to take all my clothes and belongings with me to the ultra sound room. Again, I felt awkward. I had to walk from X-ray through two waiting areas with sock feet wearing one of those stupid gowns. A couple of people in the waiting areas looked at me as I was rushing about. I felt like saying, "Haven't you ever seen a hurried, awkward, overwhelmed woman jog through a waiting room in a flimsly gown and black socks before?" I arrived successfully at the ultra sound location and sat down in a chair in front of the room with all my belongings. As soon as I sat down, I realized I had forgotten my eyeglasses in the change room. Once again, I rushed through the same path back to X-ray in the stupid flimsy gown and retrieved my glasses. I was so embarrassed to be rushing around dressed like that. No one else was, just me. Back to the chair in the ultra sound hallway and as I sat and waited for my turn, I wondered why the technician wanted me so quickly as I had to wait a half hour on him. The ultra sound did not take long and once finished I hurried over to the lab for the blood work. It was another late finish that day, and I was so anxious to get out of there I practically ran out of the building. The best part of leaving that day was I had no more appointments there. I was done! Thank God!

I did have to go to a different Vancouver hospital for a bone density scan the next day. It was Debbie's day off, so Terry, she and I went together. At the nuclear medicine department, they gave me the radioactive and this time I had to wait two hours before they could give me the scan. During that time, the three of us went for lunch and shopping. I really enjoyed spending my time with them. Once back at the hospital I loved the scan. It took about one hour and I was so relaxed I woke myself up more than once with a quiet snore. I did not want this scan to end.

The room was darkened and I felt secure inside this machine. I was not to move a muscle, having to be perfectly still throughout the entire scan. Again I thought about all the recent events. I thought about my family and thought about God. I took this time to consider a family meeting when I got home and thought about everything I had to say to them. Yes, this was a great idea. From that point I was anxious to have the meeting, but now was the time to enjoy this quiet time.

Before my flight down to Vancouver I made arrangements to go to Vancouver Island and stay a couple days with Lydia. Terry and Debbie dropped me off at the ferry terminal and Randal's sister, my sister-in-law Donna picked me up at the other side. It was good to see Ladysmith again. I moved there after my first marriage ended. I bought a quaint 1600 square foot home for me and the kids. It had four bedrooms, so we all had our own room. From Ladysmith I was able to commute to the university in Nanaimo. It was a good time in my life. The backyard was small and had no grass. I didn't want to plant a lawn, so I hired a handsome handyman to put gravel rocks down. I ended up marrying that handsome handyman. Those days were some of my happiest. Randal and I really had something special.

I was very happy to see Lydia again. We gave each other a big hug and began our time together. Jean graced us with her presence by coming to visit us from Victoria. It was good to talk with her and hear her stories about treatment. Since my birthday is in April, Lydia made me my favourite supper, steak. Lydia made a seafood dish for her and Jean. The three of us sat down in the living room with T.V. trays enjoying an excellent supper and we watched an old Kirk Douglas movie. I often think about how special that evening was. That evening I received a phone call from my other brother, Bryan who also lives on the Island, in Duncan.

I had planned to spend Friday and Saturday night with Lydia and take the ferry back to the mainland with Bryan and Delphine on Sunday. When Bryan phoned me, he wanted me to spend Saturday night with them. I could not. I had promised Lydia I would stay at her house and she was looking forward to it. I didn't want to change my plans. I didn't want to disappoint my brother either, so I spent Saturday evening at their house. While at Bryan's house we had a ball. Bryan owns bongo drums and jams with a band on weekends. He took out a tamborine and handed it to me. Delphine played some of her old records from the 60's and 70's on an old turntable. While the music played Bryan bongoed on his drums, Delphine played the maracas and I sang while tapping the tamborine. We were having a blast! It felt so good to be with them at their home. I never used to feel that way - took it for granted, but now I revelled in it. It was a special evening I'll always remember! They drove me back to Ladysmith at 11:00 pm.

The time I spent with Lydia, Jean, Bryan and Delphine was precious. Since cancer entered my life I woke up in many different ways. True appreciation for the people God has given to me is paramount. Each person is so unique and so too is my relationships with them. I just appreciate everyone so much more than I did before. This is what life is for - loving God and each other. *"Love the Lord your God with all your heart and with all your soul and with all your mind and with all your strength... Love your neighbor as yourself. There is no greater command than these." (Matthew12:30-31)*

The next morning arrived with a ton of snow, something very unusual for Vancouver Island in April. I woke up early and when I came out of my room, Lydia was playing cards at her dining room table while enjoying her morning coffee - a morning ritual she has been enjoying for years. Behind her I could see the wintery scene through the sliding glass doors. All I could say was, "Oh, no way!" I knew instantly my brother Bryan would be in a frantic state of mind. I wasn't out of bed five minutes when he telephoned me. With urgency in his voice he strongly suggested we take the ferry to Terry and Debbie's house the next day. Debbie was planning a big supper meal for me for my birthday that day. My nephew and his wife were coming from out of town to see me. I had to show up. I calmed Bryan down, so I thought, and talked him into going to the mainland that morning, snow or no snow.

For people living in the north, snow is rarely a factor that prevents people from driving to daily activities and responsibilities. We have snow in the north for at least eight months - no, about ten months out of the year accompanied by -15 to-40 C temperatures. Schools remain open, as does everything else. Our roads are not ploughed as they are on Vancouver Island and the lower mainland. The main roads usually have snow on them, but pavement is visible where the tires wear down the snow. Residential roads are rarely cleared. Snow and packed ice are the norm. Parking lots are never cleared either. People drive in these road conditions everyday up here. Such panic down south when it snows! I knew exactly how this Vancouver Island snowfall would turn out. I knew the snow would be almost gone by noon, but I did understand Bryan. I used to panic too when I lived on the Island. When I saw a snowflake in the air I would immediately drive home and stay home. I never ventured out until the roads were clear, which was never very long. I got my way. Bryan and I solidified our plans that morning at 7:30 am.

At 8:00 I was sitting at the dining room table with Lydia, and by this time Jean had woken up and joined us. I was enjoying a cup of coffee and finishing my make-up when Bryan pulled into the driveway. Bryan sent Delphine to come into the house to get me. I sympathized with Delphine because I knew Bryan was in a panic, and in turn put her into a panic. She asked me why I wasn't ready yet. I was floored. I knew they were coming sometime in the morning, but I didn't realize they were practically out the door after our phone call. Knowing how my brother was feeling I very quickly got dressed and packed. I wasn't returning to Lydia's house before flying back to the north, so I made sure I had everything with me. We were on the road to the ferry 15 minutes after they pulled into the driveway.

We were merrily driving down the highway, which by now was almost clear, enjoying our time together. We arrived at the Nanaimo ferry terminal and had only two hours to wait for the ferry! As we sat in the van waiting and chatting, Bryan's cell phone rang. It was my husband phoning with bad news. Lydia phoned him and told him I had forgotten my purse at her house. The previous night when Bryan dropped me off at Lydia's I had put my purse down at the front door, a location I rarely used. That morning we exited out the back door, so I did not see it on my way out. I had been so rushed and concerned about getting out the door, my purse didn't even cross my mind. Unfortunately, my purse contained my I.D., which I needed for my flight home. There was no way I could have Lydia mail it to me. We knew we had to go back to Lydia's house and retrieve my forgotten purse. Bryan had to drive out of the short-line up, get his money back, and we drove back to Ladysmith. It was good to see Lydia again, as I could not give her a proper goodbye the first time I left. It was important to me that she knew how much I appreciated everything she did for me. My jaw almost dropped when Delphine asked me, "How could you forget your purse?" I looked at her and calmly stated, "I was rushed." We travelled the now clear highway back to the ferry. We caught the ferry and arrived safely at Terry's house in Mission.

Another great evening at Terry's home. It was comforting to have both my brothers and their families with me. Debbie made a superb meal and we all sat around enjoying being together. Bryan had brought some of his instruments and we "jammed." My nephew's son and daughter were absolutely priceless. Both of them were under the age of five and jammed along with everyone. It was another wonderful experience that I will always remember. Family isn't always perfect and smooth, and that is why we experience truly beautiful times like this, to ease away the tougher times.

I enjoyed a couple of quiet days with Terry and Debbie before flying back to Fort St. John. They were so good to me. Terry driving me all the way into Vancouver three times and patiently waiting for me. Debbie had given me a beautiful breast cancer angel and a wonderful book about healing one's hurts. Debbie putting on a great family get together for my birthday. Terry allowing me to watch some of his satellite T.V. while missing some of his sports. Both of them were so positive and they lifted my spirits. What I appreciated the most was their example of living a content and positive life despite the great loss within their family. I learned some important lessons during my week's stay with them and I am fortunate they are a part of my family. I thank God for them.

As I previously explained, Debbie and I were able to share our personal experiences with each other. The exchanging of our stories and some of the familiar aspects we share strengthened me. I told her about my three - year depression and the suicide I planned. I told her about my "fear of flying" and the young boy on the T.V. I explained how my depression had been transformed into a positive attitude, a fighting spirit and a sense of adventure. I told her that through God's ways I knew I had more years left to live. I confided to her about some of my family dynamics and how they contributed to my depression and anxiety. Heck, I told Debbie almost everything. It was a relief to give account of my struggles to someone outside of my immediate family and have them understand me.

I also told Debbie I was planning on having a family meeting when I got back home. I had to tell everybody about my illness, how serious it was and how serious it would continue to be. I realize they knew cancer was serious, but I felt I had to tell them just how serious it really was. I had to explain my treatment plan and what to expect from it. Most importantly, I had to explain to them what I needed and expected from each one of them in the coming months. Debbie agreed it was important to establish my expectations and boundaries. I let Debbie know how her and Terry had positively influenced me and how much I needed that. I almost didn't want to leave, but I knew I could take this positive experience with me and draw upon it whenever I needed to do so.

It felt great to see Randal waiting at the airport for me. After retrieving my luggage we started on our way home. Once in the truck, Randal told me he had seen Dr. Thomson while I was in Mission. He had mentioned this to me on the phone, but now went into greater detail. Dr. Thomson told Randal that my chemotherapy was the strongest dosage they have ever had at our hospital. I was shocked and wondered, "Wow, how sick am I?" I had an appointment with Dr. Thomson that same day and I had many questions for him.

Dr. Thomson was his usual pleasant self when I saw him. He had all the information from the oncologist. The first thing Dr. Thomson told me was my dosage of chemo was the strongest this hospital had ever had. He told me about the side effects. He told me how the chemo will cause body aches and the medication to enhance my white blood cell count will also cause body aches "It's going to be a rough go of it, but I'm keen if you are." "Oh I'm keen!" I felt positive about having chemotherapy. Of course I had fears about how sick I would become, but my sense of adventure gave me strength. I was very eager to begin chemo; I could hardly wait. I was feeling fantastic and then Dr. Thomson said something that put an end to my great mood. "Without any treatment you have a 40 -50 percent, but we're going to build on that. We're going to bring it up to 80 percent." Without treatment 40 -50 percent! I couldn't get my mind off that sentence, 40 -50 percent! That's not very much. Oh God, why did this have to happen?

I got into the truck to drive home and just sat there and thought, "40 -50 percent. That's not very much. That's not very good!" Suddenly fear encompassed me and I was once again terrified. I continued to just sit in the truck and be frightened and sad. Tears ran down my cheeks as I feared my mortality. Oh God, not now, please not now. As I drove home I thought about everything Dr. Thomson said, especially the 40 -50 percent, and the tears impaired my vision. I forced myself to stop crying. I ordered myself to be strong. I reminded myself of God's ways. I was a few hours away from the family meeting and I had to get it together. I did.

That evening my family and I were sitting in my living room when I began my "speech". I put up a good front for everyone. I told everyone to please be quiet and listen. I let them know that when I was finished it would be their turn to talk. I was doing a rather fine job as they listened. I described the positive experience I had at Terry's house. I told them how supportive and positive they were and how much that helped me with my own attitude. I told everyone if they had anything negative to say about each other that I was no longer the person to talk to about it. Any issues they had with each other had to be between them and not include me. Randal would have to be the only breadwinner, so he was not expected to do any household cleaning. Matt and Melissa were expected to do the housekeeping when I would be too sick to do it myself - no arguments. Nick and Mom were expected to help out when asked. I needed everyone to be as positive as possible in order for me to stay positive. I didn't expect perfection and realized there would still be issues. I just needed everyone to work out their issues peacefully.

In addition, I felt it was very important to explain to everybody that this was my cancer. I was going to be the one in charge of my treatment including any decisions regarding my treatment. No one was to compare me to any other cancer patients, "Everyone's cancer is different, as is their treatment. This is my cancer and this is my treatment. I will make all the decisions regarding my treatment as this is my body and I know it better than anyone else. I do value everyone's opinion, but all decisions will be mine to make." I began to cry as I described how scared I felt, but kept it together before ending my talk.

I was very proud of all of them. They all sat quietly and listened. They all said they would respect my wishes and be positive. They agreed to keep family issues peaceful. They asked questions about my treatment plan, the drugs, the side effects and how they could help. Randal had a great idea to make me fruit shakes. Mom offered to come over and help with housekeeping. The kids made it clear they understood when asked to do something - do it. My tests were complete, I had my treatment plan and I had the support of my family behind me. I was ready for my next step - chemotherapy.

My Descent into Chemotherapy

For your namesake; O Lord
Preserve my life;
In your righteousness bring me out
Of trouble. (Psalm 143:11)

Cycle One

Two days before my first chemotherapy cycle, I had to go to the hospital to meet with one of the chemo nurses to discuss my treatment. Once at the hospital I was feeling a little nervous, but also equally excited. I made my way to the chemotherapy department and when I walked in I was more than surprised. It was not much bigger than a breadbox. In reality it was the size of an office. This one room consisted of two recliners, one desk, a portable wall of patient charts, two small chairs for others and various other medical necessities. Both nurses were there, Janice and Virginia, along with an older woman receiving her chemotherapy. Her husband was sitting in a chair beside her and I remember thinking, "How nice for her to have such a faithful supporter." It was an independent thought for her; no judgment or comparison towards my husband. I felt a little uncomfortable and awkward walking in, but that feeling was quickly dashed by the warm smiles from everyone.

The atmosphere was warm and welcoming due to the pleasantness and consideration of Janice and Virginia. Janice, 15 years my senior, immediately introduced herself, as did Virginia, about 15 years my junior. It was not difficult to notice Janice's pretty face nicely framed by her shoulder length blonde hair. Janice's soft appearance and pleasant attitude immediately put me at ease. It was not difficult to notice Virginia's young attractive face and her hourglass figure beautifully highlighted by her scrubs. I envied Virginia's youth and envied both nurses for their health. After all the proper and professional introductions, Janice suggested we go to a different room for my appointment as privacy did not exist in the Breadbox.

As I followed Janice down the hallways, I concentrated on clearing my mind from any nervous thoughts, so I could best understand all the information I was going to hear. Although still a little nervous, I was enjoying the sense of adventure that filled my spirit. Janice led me into an empty patient room and we grabbed a couple of chairs and sat side by side. Janice began by confirming my chemo dosage was the strongest they had ever had at the hospital and confirmed the name of the drugs. She also confirmed my hair would fall out - will definitely fall out. Losing my hair did not concern me the least bit. I was looking forward to it. I planned on having fun with wigs. Most importantly Janice explained the side effects in greater detail.

Janice concentrated most of her time on nausea. She explained exactly what nausea was. I listened as she described nausea as an upset stomach, vomiting, loss of appetite, and a sense of feeling full. She told me if I vomit even just once I was to go to the hospital immediately. She told me once vomiting occurs, it is very difficult to get under control. This would cause me to have to stay in the hospital until all vomiting ceased. Nausea was my biggest concern regarding chemotherapy. I have been sensitive to nausea ever since my three pregnancies. Each pregnancy put me in bed for months due to morning sickness. Actually, I didn't have morning sickness - I suffered from 24 hour sickness. The only relief I was able to find was when I slept. However, knowing about chemotherapy and nausea prepared me mentally, but I hoped the nausea would not be a problem this time.

Janice then explained about the importance of drinking water. As with all chemo patients I had to drink at least two litres of water daily. I wondered how I was going to be able to drink so much. She explained the water is very important because it carries the chemo throughout the entire body. Therefore, the chemo would be able to get into all the nooks and crannies and do its job the best it can. Janice explained any nausea I experienced would prevent me from drinking the water - impairing the effectiveness of the chemo.

Other side effects Janice mentioned were allergic reaction, fatigue, mouth sores, diarrhea, burning urination, constipation, metallic taste, increased bleeding, vein damage, and pain affecting my joints and/or muscles. At this point Janice explained the drug Neupogen that I would be taking to boost my white blood cell count in the bone marrow. She explained this would cause me pain, as Dr. Thomson said it would as well. Because of my strong chemo dosage, I had to take it. I was to inject myself with the Neupogen for seven days following my treatment. Janice also told me I had to take my temperature daily as fever is an indicator of infection. It was important not to get an infection or contract any illness, as this would put my health in peril as well as delay chemo. I didn't want any delays!

Janice gave me the protocol I was to follow before I would be able to receive my chemo. She gave me a green medical card with a yellow dot on it. This card was to be used every time I had to go to the hospital. She also gave me my paper order for the bloodwork to be done the following day. This paper also had a yellow dot on it. Everytime I had to go to the hospital for bloodwork I had to go straight to Admitting and give them the green card with the yellow dot. The yellow dot meant "cancer" and gave me priority over all the other patients. I was to follow the same procedure at the lab and at the doctor's office. Remember how important it is not to be exposed to illness of any sort. Janice joked and said it was like having a VIP card. I thought this was great! Too bad I had to get cancer to be considered a VIP. I couldn't wait to try it out!

Janice explained everything with absolute clarity. I was impressed by her knowledge and her kind nature. She answered any lingering questions I had. It was a positive and pleasant meeting and I felt very confident towards the care I was going to receive. At the meeting's end Janice escorted me to the elevator. As we were walking I concluded she was an excellent nurse and I wondered how we would get along throughout the course of my treatment. As I went down to the main floor I was excited and anxious to begin my chemotherapy treatment.

The first day of my chemotherapy finally arrived, April 30, 2008. Yes, I was very excited and anxious to get my injection. When I speak about my sense of adventure I knew it would not be a glorious, joy filled, wonderous, exciting and fun period of time excempt of pain, suffering, depression, heart ache, frustration and sadness. All adventures are composed of both positive and negative. It's like everything else in life; one must accept the negative as it is part and parcel a part of all experiences. I was just so happy to be finally getting down to the nitty gritty of my battle with breast cancer. On this day I was devoid of anxiety and fear. I trusted In God - He had my life in His hands. ***"The Lord will sustain him on his sickbed and restore him from his bed of illness." (Psalm 41:3)***

As Randal and I walked into the Breadbox my day became even happier in a snap. There in one of the recliners sat Leah. Both Leah and I were so surprised to see each other. Leah commented, "Wow! You look great." I really did look considerably better since our last meeting in the hospital. I was glad Leah could see how I really looked. I felt redeemed from my previous frightful appearance. Leah was being treated for a condition unrelated to cancer. I took a seat in the other recliner while Randal took a chair across from me. It felt great as I settled my body in the shape of the chair. I was ready to descend into the abyss of chemotherapy.

I had been told by both doctors and nurses what to expect along the way of my descent. Now I was about to experience chemotherapy first hand. While Janice was at the desk tending to administrative duties, Virginia began attending to me. She placed my right arm in an electric heating pad to prepare my veins for the I.V. Randal and Leah were conversing while Virginia inserted the shunt for the I.V. I am terribly squeamish about such procedures, so I turned my head until it was in my vein. Virginia began with the anti nausea-drug and I prayed I would not suffer from nausea and vomiting.

It didn't take long for the drug to drip to completion. Afterwards Virginia brought out the big guns. Two huge syringes filled with red liquid, "the red stuff". I was surprised by the size and amount and equally surprised by how it was administered. It was injected manually instead of dripping through the I.V.. It was a slow process. It took about 20 -30 minutes. While Virginia continued to administer the chemo I began to pray inside myself, "Please God let this poison do its job. Let this be okay. Please don't let me get nausea. Please be with me." I visualized the chemo as an army of pac mans aggressively hunting down the known enemy - the cancer cells, and destroying them. As each pac man destroyed a cancer cell the yellow warrior grew more powerful. I felt very comfortable during this process. I was happy and relaxed and enjoying everyone's company.

Once the red stuff was finished Virginia put the second bag of chemo on the I.V.. As it began to drip down I muted out all the voices in the Breadbox and again visualized the army of pac mans soldiering throughout my body hunting and destroying the enemy. Great company and conversation continued between everyone in the Breadbox. At one point Randal asked

Janice about chemo and why some people lose their hair and others do not. Janice explained there are over 300 different types of chemo and some do not cause hair loss. I was pleased to find this out because so many people tried to comfort me by saying I might not lose my hair. I wanted to lose my hair. I prepared myself for this. "It better fall out or I'll be mad," I thought to myself numerous times.

Other interesting topics filled the air as I sat enjoying this experience. After the second bag was completely empty I was given a saline rinse. The entire process took about four hours. Before leaving, Janice mentioned it usually takes five hours for any nausea to occur and reminded me what to do if it did. Both Janice and Virginia are very serious about their jobs and truly care about their patients. Janice is equally serious about nausea and I can appreciate that!

At the end of my first chemo cycle Randal and I went out for lunch. I had a healthy appetite. I ordered my favorite, a cheeseburger with fries and gravy - and a coke of course. This was to be my last coke as I knew it was not allowed while on chemo unless I doubled my water intake. I wasn't about to do that! As Randal and I ate our lunch I felt fantastic. I hoped I would remain feeling this good. I was happy Randal came to my first treatment with me and happy he took me out for lunch. I felt his support. Marriage is funny. Just when you think your husband doesn't care, he does something thoughtful and caring.

After our lunch, Randal dropped me off at home and then went to the pharmacy to get my prescriptions filled. When he came home he told me how expensive my anti-nausea drug was - $5.00 a pill. We both had sticker shock. It reminded me of the time Randal, Matt, Melissa and myself had immunizations before leaving for Korea. Randal and the kids received three shots and because I was behind in my inoculations I received four. Once the injections were completed it came time to pay. It cost a staggering $500.00! I'm sure my jaw hit the floor - $500.00 for inoculations! That's one half of $1,000.00! For inoculations! I reluctantly took the cash out of my purse and almost cried when I handed it over to the nurse. Once we were in the car I told Randal I needed a drink - $500.00 for inoculations - that's unreal! We were fortunate this time, as Randal's job had medical benefits, so we did not have to pay $5.00 a pill. However, the cost of one particular drug would soon knock us out.

I watched our owl clock on the wall tick away. On the fifth hour since my chemo I still had no nausea. I was so relieved. The day shifted into evening and still no nausea. I was very restless though. I became very restless during the night. I could not sleep. I stayed awake all night. There was nothing but junk on T.V. and I didn't feel like doing anything because I was so restless. When morning came I told Randal about my night. He didn't know what to do about it any more than I did. The bright side was I still felt very healthy - until I received a phone call from Virginia.

The previous day while at the Breadbox, Janice had phoned the pharmacy to order the Neupogen. Virginia phoned to tell me I had to begin my injections this day. She also explained the hospital pharmacy does not carry the drug. I had to go to a public pharmacy to get it. I didn't think this was a big deal until she told me how much this would cost me. She bravely stated it would cost me $1,200.00. I was speechless. The inoculations paled in comparison to this. I didn't know what to do. We didn't have the money and I needed the drug.

In hysterics I phoned Randal at work. He was equally as shocked as I was. We were at a loss of what to do. We both knew I needed the drug because of the strong chemo dosage. My white blood cells (WBC) would definitely take a dramatic decline and delay future cycles. Randal said he would phone our pharmacy to see if his benefits plan would cover the cost. Just as I hung up the phone, Virginia phoned back and suggested I phone the B.C. Cancer Agency to find out if they cover the cost of this drug.

I spoke to a pleasant woman from the Vancouver Cancer Agency and she explained the agency does not cover the cost of this medication because they would go bankcrupt if they did. "So would I." I felt like saying. This lady suggested I contact the Canadian Cancer Society. I spoke to another pleasant woman and she made an appointment to come to our house and see if they could help us. I then phoned the B.C. Medical Services Plan. Being 44 years of age, I have heard my share of B.S., but this was something else. The B.C. medical does not cover the cost of this drug because it is not considered a cancer-fighting drug! It is not a cancer fighting drug, yet I could not fight my cancer without it! They did however give me the number to phone Pharmacare. Again I spoke to a pleasant woman and she told me she would mail me an application. Yes, Pharmacare would cover the cost of this drug after we paid a 2,500.00 deductable! I felt so defeated. It is stressful enough battling cancer; one does not need more financial stress on top of it. Randal came home from work at lunch and told me his benefits plan does not cover the drug. I told him about the B.C. Cancer Agency, B.C. Medical, Canadian Cancer Society, and Pharmacare. We were sunk.

After lunch Janice phoned to tell me she spoke to a pharmacist near the hospital. He agreed to give me the drug and we could make payments on it. She also told me the drug actually cost $1,200.00 each week! That made a grand total of $4,800.00! I was even more shocked than before! How were we going to pay for this drug? I went to the bank and withdrew $700.00 and went to pick up the Neupogen. With great resentment I went to the hospital and Virginia taught me how to inject myself. I resented everything. I resented the fact I had cancer, I resented the fact I had a breast removed, I resented the fact I had to have chemotherapy, I resented the fact I could not work, I resented the fact we had more financial stress, and I resented the fact this drug I needed cost so damn much.

The following day, Laura the helpful woman from the Canadian Cancer Society came to our house and we went over all our finances with her. It didn't take long to find out the CCS does not pay for the cost of drugs. Shit! The following week we received our application from Pharmacare. We mailed it back the same week and hoped for the best. Pharmacare processed our application at a snail's pace and in the meantime we continued to make payments on the drug. By the time Pharmacare approved our application we had already paid $4,200.00 of our own money. Very frustrating. I chose to look at the bright side of this situation. I was able to receive the drug and had zero delays with my chemo.

Two days after my first chemo I began to feel the effects. Apart from the restlessness the first side effect I felt was a strange and irritating sensation in my head. I called it "chemo haze". I then started to feel fatigue and body aches. I also had a headache that refused to go away, and the Neupogen made my body feel heavy. All I could do was lie on the couch. My little kitty Mia would not leave my side. She got as close to me as possible. She found a nice little spot between my neck and shoulders. It was so sweet and she made me feel cared for. She stayed with me for hours.

During the night, as my family slept peacefully, I became extremely restless and fatigued. I was up, down and all around. I could not get comfortable no matter where I put my body. I tried to relax in the recliner, the couch and attempted a few times to lie in bed. I would only be comfortable for about ten minutes and then I was on the move again. I watched some T.V. for a while, but there was only junk on again. I played some computer games, but my body would become too restless to remain in the chair. I tried reading and again would become restless. Then I tried to watch T.V., then computer games, and on and on this went throughout the entire night. The only bright spot during this was that I could spend some time with Randal and the kids before they went to work and school. After they left the house I climbed in bed at 9 am and finally fell asleep. I would wake up at 3:00 pm. This continued throughout the weekend and into the next week. Randal was at a loss as to how to help me, so he went to speak to Janice about it. Janice arranged a meeting for the three of us the next day.

Before leaving the house to go to the hospital to see Janice, Randal noticed I did not have anything to eat. He suggested I eat something, but I didn't have an appetite. I grabbed some soda crackers and took them with me. We arrived at the Breadbox and after all the usual pleasantries Janice sat me down in one of the recliners. She sat facing me. She had a pen and paper in her hands and asked me to tell her everything I was experiencing. I began with describing body aches, especially in my feet. It felt like I had no meat on my soles; like I was walking on bone. I then went on to describe how restless I was, especially at night. Randal interjected, "She's all over the place." I added in addition to restlessness, I feel anxious, always anxious. I mentioned the nagging headache and admitted it was getting worse. Janice wrote everything down as I described it. Janice suggested Ativan (Lorazepam) for the anxiety, and Percacets (Oxycodone) for the pain. She then phoned my doctor and he ordered the prescriptions in for me at our drug store. That fast!

I was feeling rather fine during our meeting. Janice was kind and understanding and then the subject of water came up, "Okay, how much water are you drinking?" Before I could get the words out of my mouth Randal tattled on me, "Oh, she might be drinking half the amount she should be." I knew right away I was in trouble. Janice didn't say a word about the water, but she looked me in the eye and asked, "Are you experiencing any nausea?" "No I'm feeling fine." Janice looked at the soda crackers resting on my lap and quietly asked, "So why the crackers?" I thought, "Why does this woman have to be so smart? I should have known better." I told her I just didn't feel very hungry. As earlier stated, Janice takes her job very seriously and does exceedingly well at it. I was about to experience this first hand.

"Do you remember at our first meeting how I explained what was considered nausea?" I told her I remember. "Do you remember when I said feeling full or a loss of appetite is considered nausea?" "Yes, I remember." Janice put her hand on my knee and with kindness asked, "So are you experiencing any nausea?" I was stubborn and didn't want to admit it, but I replied, "I guess I am." I was angry I had nausea! Janice, in her kind professional manner, reminded me of the importance of water and how the nausea prevents me from drinking it. I clearly understood. She told me to increase the anti nausea drug and start drinking my water. Point taken, Janice, and well done! The meeting was over and we left for home.

As Randal and I travelled down the elevator I was feeling a wee bit scolded, but I quickly got over that. From that day on I did exactly what I was told to do. My medical team was doing what was expected of them. I had to have faith and trust the expertise of these educated and experienced practitioners - they were guiding me through this treatment for the benefit of my health and life. I owed it to them, my family and myself to do what was expected of me. Four days prior to my second cycle I began to feel better. The day of my second cycle I drove myself to the hospital. I was feeling great!

Cycle Two

I was free of nervousness and anxiety as I made my way to the Breadbox for my second chemo cycle. When I walked in, Janice was at the desk and there was a woman in one of the recliners. This woman looked to be very close to my age. I said "Hello" to everyone and they returned my greeting. I sat down in the other recliner and Janice prepared my arm for the I.V. with the heating pad again. I was happy to tell Janice how much better I was feeling. The Ativan calmed me down and I could finally get comfortable and sleep. The Percacets helped with the body aches and took my headache away completely. Virginia was not working that day. She had gone back east to work on her wedding preparations. While Janice waited for my veins to be ready, she spoke to the other patient. This patient seemed like a positive woman and I was anxious to talk to her.

As Janice began the procedure of hooking me up to the I.V. she continued to speak to the other patient. I waited for an opportunity to interject in their conversation. When the opportunity arose I jumped right in. I then introduced myself and she told me her name was Teresa. Janice had the I.V. completed and soon the anti-nausea drug was dripping nicely. I continued to talk to Teresa. I liked her instantly. She was a down-to-earth and pleasant type. As we talked, Janice began to inject the red stuff once the anti nausea drug had finished dripping. Janice joined our conversation. It was so good to have a woman I could relate to - to talk to, and have Janice there to educate me even more about cancer and chemotherapy.

Teresa was a small woman and due to her hair loss she wore a kerchief on her head. She called it her "do rag". I thought that name was unusual, but cute. Teresa had a great sense of humor, which made me feel at ease and happy. She shared her story with me and I shared mine with her. I really envied her that day because it was her second-to-last treatment. She would be starting her radiation soon. I was so jealous. She was almost done and I was just beginning. Teresa commented on my hair and asked me how I felt about losing it. I told her I never felt sad about it and told her about the wig Jean mailed to me. I also told her I had bought two more wigs. I admitted I was actually looking forward to losing my hair.

At that point Janice told us a hilarious story about one of her former patients. This lady had long beautiful hair and the thought of losing it was unimaginable to her. This lady had convinced herself, despite Janice's warnings, that her hair would not fall out. One day this lady and her husband was outside when the weather turned windy. Before she knew it the wind had blown her hair right off her head. She was now completely bald. She was also heartbroken. Janice told us this woman was very traumatized by her hair loss. I took this time to tell Janice and Teresa that is how I felt about my left breast.

Teresa did not have to have a mastectomy. She had two tumors removed and had three lymph nodes that were positive for cancer. She revealed how disfigured she felt. I was relieved to know I was not alone with feelings of disfigurement. Having one breast is unnatural and has profoundly affected my sense of being a woman and a wife. When I feel sad about it I think of the day I will have my reconstruction. Teresa noticed I had two breasts and asked me if I had a prosthesis. I explained I refused to pay $400.00 for a prosthesis. I had purchased two breast enhancers years ago that I never used. I described them and told her they were in my bra. Teresa was very curious about them, so I reached inside my bra, pulled one out and handed it to her. She remarked how natural it felt, so Janice wanted to hold it too. The three of us giggled and I told them how I had caught my kids playing with them when I left them sitting on the coffee table. Teresa and Janice really laughed when I said, "My kids said they felt natural too!"

It came time for Teresa to leave and I was so disappointed to see her go. I gained so much in that short period of time from her. I couldn't watch Teresa walk out that door without knowing I might never see her again. I boldly asked her if we could exchange phone numbers. We did and I looked forward to future conversations with her. Not so long after Teresa left, my treatment was finished. It went by so fast because of the good company and the positive atmosphere.

When I came home I did some housework and started the laundry. I knew I had at least two days to get things done before the side effects kicked in. I was apprehensive about the onset of the side effects as I knew they would become worse. Knowing they were going to be worse, I concluded it would be useless to worry about it. I made the decision to concentrate on other matters. Through the grace of God I still had a positive attitude and fighting spirit. More importantly I still had His promise to be with me every moment helping me.

During the first few days my family life was business as usual. The kids went to school and work, and Randal, of course, continued to go to work. At the end of his shift he came home and did whatever necessary to help me. He also came home on his lunch hour. I enjoyed his company and hearing stories about his company's work politics. Also during these days he was able to take care of any needs I had. My mom came over and did some light housekeeping. It was good to have her around.

My side effects kicked in right on schedule. During the afternoon of day three after my treatment, I noticed "chemo haze". I really hated this sensation. The chemo haze was worse. I hoped it would not last too long. At least this time I did not have a headache, and if I did, I had something to take for it that worked. Only hours after noticing the chemo haze, other side effects began to follow.

The next side effect to arrive was the body pain. As the day progressed so too did the pain. I could feel the pain in my feet again. Oh, how it hurt! The anxiety and restlessness was next. As with the other side effects, the anxiety and restlessness was worse. I took the Ativan and it really helped. During this cycle I developed a new side effect, heatburn. It was not too bad and it was easily taken care of with simple name brand tablets. Randal purchased some liquid medication to also help with the heartburn. As the burning intensified throughout the coming days, I drank more liquid antacid. I had hearburn almost every day of this cycle.

I followed the same routine for all my cycles. Every second Tuesday morning I went to the hospital with my yellow dotted green card and had my bloodwork done. Next I would go see Dr. Thomson for my check up and get my prescriptions. Then I went to the pharmacy. Then I would come home and carefully put all my pills in the pill box my mom gave me, and put my $1,200.00 supply of Neupogen in the fridge. I would spend the remainder of my day getting laundry done, sweeping, cleaning the kitchen, dusting and performing some other duties I knew would not get done until the Tuesday before my next cycle. Every second Wednesday I would go to the Breadbox to have my chemo, and come home. After a day or two the side effects arrived and the routine would happen all over again.

By Friday evening my side effects were all present. For a while I would be in the living room with Randal laying on the couch with Mia right beside me. There came a point when I became far too fatigued and restless to remain on the couch. When I got to this point, I would go to the bathroom and take my antacid, anti-nausea pills, two percacets, one Ativan and one muscle relaxant, and then up to my bed. It wasn't necessarily late. Sometimes I went to bed at 7:00 or 8:00pm. Randal thought this was great because he could watch any old stupid show on T.V.

Every night I slowly trudged up my steep staircase with my body and feet aching all the way. I would climb up on my bed as awkward as an elephant. Once in bed I would let out a deep sigh usually followed by, "Oh God." I would remain in the same position for a few moments. I would then find the remote control and try to find something worthwhile to watch. Mere minutes after getting comfortable Mia would soon be at my side. I was exhausted! Sometimes I would sleep for a few hours in the evening and have strange dreams. Most nights my legs would become so restless, so I would take another Ativan and muscle relaxant. I always had a pillow between my legs and that did help. I would eventually fall asleep around 11:00pm.

In the mornings I usually woke up anytime between 10:00am and noon, and begin my typical day. I would climb awkwardly out of my bed and get to the bathroom as fast as I could. I would gather up all the pills I was to take and drink them down with water of course. Next I would take some antacid and fill up my water jug. If Randal was home I would sit with him, and if he was at work I would sit and watch some T.V. I always waited a couple of hours after waking up before I gave myself the Neupogen injection.

As I went about my day my little Mia was always near me. Whenever I sat or lay down Mia was there. Whenever I got up to do something Mia followed me. My family and I were fascinated by how she was always either on me, beside me, near me, or snuggled into the form of my body. One day when I was quite sick I was lying on the couch and Mia hopped up on top of me. She fussed and fussed about as she tried to find a comfortable position. Randal was sitting in his recliner when I told him to look at Mia.

There was my special little kitty with all four paws on the top of my head about to lie down. How sweet - but my head?!

I believe God gave me a special little angel kitty to care for me in her own way. As long as Mia was around I was never alone. She followed me from room to room and would always wait for me. I just loved it. I loved being with my small cat cuddling with her and showing her how much I appreciated her care. Some nights she would be ready to go to bed before me. She would sit at the bottom of the staircase and look at me. I would say to her, "Not now, Mia. It's too early." She would come back over to me, lie down beside me and patiently wait a little longer. Whenever Mia and I were on my bed she wouldn't allow any of the other cats up. Mia considered me hers and I never had such a faithful little nurse.

As time passed during cycle two, my side effects worsened, but the chemo haze started to ease off and eventually it was gone. The heartburn became worse - a lot worse. I spent the best part of my weekend drinking antacid. As soon as Monday morning came I was sitting in my doctor's office at exactly 9 am. He gave me some acid reflux pills and told me to increase my water. How fantastic - more water! The pills he gave me only helped a little, but whenever I felt that burn I drank water until I felt better. I noticed at this time I could no longer eat dairy products. Milk is my favorite beverage and I was so disappointed I could no longer drink it. However, I could still eat eggs and a small amount of cheese. Dealing with the side effects was proving difficult and soon I was right back in the doctor's office.

Tuesday evening I recognized the symptoms of something every woman dreads - the much detested yeast infection. I wanted this fixed as quickly as humanly possible, but this was not what sent me to the doctor. Wednesday morning I promptly purchased medication for the yeast infection. The next morning when I woke up I instantly noticed there was something wrong with my left eye. It was very red. I was angry because I knew this was an eye infection. Once again I was at the doctor's office at 9 am. By this time I noticed the side effects were beginning to diminish.

The weekend arrived and I could feel my body recovering from the chemo. I felt good enough to get out of the house, so Mom and I went shopping at the mall. Oh how great it was to get out of my house. Heck, it was great to get out of my housecoat! Mom and I went to all our favorite stores, and some not so favorite stores. My mom, always worrying about me asked, "Are you sure you're not overdoing it?" I explained to her staying at home would be overdoing it. It is so important to get out and do something when good health permits. Even just a walk around the block helps. My mom treated me to a nice lunch. I noticed my mouth felt different, but I put it out of my mind, thinking it was nothing. We stayed out all Saturday afternoon and when I came home I felt really good.

Monday morning my mouth felt horrible. I looked at the inside of my mouth in the mirror and could easily see five mouth sores. I was disappointed in myself for not remembering about this side effect, but forgetting is common for chemo patients. "Chemo brain" - another wonderful side effect! Once again I was at the doctor's office at 9 am to get a prescription for these sores. I hoped this would be the end of side effects because my next cycle was only two days away. At the end of my second cycle I can honestly say I felt physically fantastic, and my emotions were holding up very well. My anxiety was nicely controlled by the Ativan. I did not have any depression, and still had a positive attitude. All that being said, I had yet to experience the worst of chemo.

Cycle Three

"Chemo Day" again. Before I left to go to the hospital I groomed myself as usual. I took great care putting on my make up, something I've always enjoyed doing. I unwrapped the towel from my head, applied my styling gel and styled my hair as usual. I put on some flattering clothes and was pleased by my appearance. I went to the kitchen and ate a healthy breakfast. I gathered up my purse and keys and decided to use the bathroom before leaving the house. I saw my reflection in the mirror and was stunned by what I saw. My hair looked terrible. It had completely flattened out. I ran my fingers through my hair and noticed a few strands of hair in my hands. I knew I would lose my hair before the day was over.

I arrived at the Breadbox where Janice and Virginia were busy working. To my great delight there was Leah in one of the recliners. Again we were happy to see each other. Janice set about to begin my I.V. and soon we were all chatting. As before, the anti nausea drug dripped to completion then Janice injected the red stuff into me. Janice took this time to ask me how I felt after my last cycle and I was happy to tell her no nausea, but I did mention the worsening hearburn. She remembered reading the side effects from all my drugs and heartburn was one of them. She gave me the same advice as Dr. Thomson. I hoped the hearburn would not be as bad this time. Soon the red stuff was done and Janice started the next chemo drip.

I relaxed in the recliner. It was so nice to be out of the house and among a great group of ladies. All four of us had so many different things to talk about. It always surprised me how rarely cancer came up in the Breadbox conversations. It was always a nice break going to the Breadbox. Cancer and chemo were always with me and when I went to the Breadbox I found a refuge there even though I was getting my chemo. The company a cancer patient finds at treatment can be the best company one could ever hope for. I always enjoyed the conversations with Janice and Virginia, and with such wonderful additions as Teresa and Leah, my chemo sessions were a relief from the hard reality of my cancer. Just like the two previous treatments this one just flew right on by, and I was disappointed when I had to leave.

When I arrived back home, I felt energetic and in good spirits. I prepared a nice supper for Randal and was anxious to tell him about my hair. When I first began my chemotherapy Randal asked me if I would let him shave off my hair when it started to fall out. I agreed. He was so anxious to do it that after my first treatment he got out the shaver when we got home. He turned on the shaver and with a sly smile said, "Okay let's go." No way did I want my hair gone that soon. I wanted to wait and see if it would fall out gradually or all at once. He was so disappointed, but I did promise he could shave it off as soon as I noticed hair loss. When Randal came home I showed him how much hair I could pull out and with another sly smile he looked at me and said, "Tonight's the night. You promised." I couldn't help but giggle.

While I was cleaning up from supper my mischievous husband made the preparations for his barbering opportunity. Randal wasn't the only one excited: I was too. I didn't have any adverse feelings about losing my hair and I had always wondered what I would look like bald. I sat down in the middle of the kitchen on a stool. Randal draped the cape around me and fired up the shaver. In his excitement he revved it up a few times and said, "Here we go!" About half way through Randal said, "Oh, that's weird." I was alarmed by his comment and wondered if I had a big dent or a protruding bone, or even worse - the number 666. I quickly snapped back, "What?!" "The way your head is shaped it looks like you have a halo." We both laughed and I said, "See! I told you I'm an angel."

After he was finished I looked down on the floor and saw all my hair. I didn't realize I had that much hair. Randal removed the cape and I ran to look in the mirror at my new look. I was so surprised. My bald head looked like everyone else's bald head. I always feared I would have an odd shaped head and if I went bald everyone would see it. I was relieved. I made Randal show me this halo he claimed I had and sure enough my bone formation did look like a halo. We decided not to say anything to Matthew and Melissa when they came home from their jobs that evening. We wanted to see the look on their faces.

Randal and I were relaxing in the living room together when Melissa came home. When walking through the kitchen I saw her and yelled out, "Hi!" She answered back, "Hi!" as she casually looked at me. Then she yelled loudly, "Oh my God Mom!" as she did a double take. She joined us in the living room and stood there just looking at me, not saying a word. I asked her if she liked my new look. She had tears in her eyes, and still didn't say a word. I tried to ease her shock and sadness by gently telling her not to cry. I did not expect this kind of reaction and was very surprised by it. I could see she had to fight the tears back and she asked me, "Why did you do that?" I explained to her how my hair had started to fall out and I wanted it shaved off. Melissa thought I should have let my hair fall out naturally and was upset by my appearance. I think it hit home for her at that moment. She did not cry in front of me, but I know my daughter. I knew she would cry when she was alone. She went upstairs to her bedroom and stayed there.

I must admit I was surprised by Melissa's reaction. Until this point Melissa kept her feelings to herself. Of course she was shocked and saddened by my diagnosis, but like her mother she maintained a positive attitude. I believe once she saw me with my bald head, the reality of the serious illness hit her. She is like me when a shocking and/or tragic situation occurs, and needs to be alone to take it all in, and like me, when she is ready to talk she does so. My daughter always puts on a brave front and she can appear as cold and uncaring. The colder and more uncaring she appears, the deeper her sadness is. I should have been more sensitive towards her that evening, but I left her alone for a couple of hours before I spoke to her about it. She's a beautiful, wonderful girl and I thank God for her life.

Matthew came home from work late in the evening and when he came into the kitchen I walked in and and, "Hi." His reaction was similar to his sister's, but he didn't have any tears. Matthew is and has always been very curious. I used to say to him, "You need to know the ins and outs of a fart." This time was no different; he was very curious. Like his sister, he wanted to know why I didn't let my hair fall out on its own. I gave him the same explanation I gave his sister. Curious, Matthew had to look at my head under a light, so he could see exactly how my head now looked. He quickly noticed there remained some little hairs - stubble. He pulled out a few hairs and was surprised by how easily they came out - effortlessly. He would pull out some hairs and say, "Oh gross!" and do it again and say, "Oh gross!" He must have done this four or five times before I made him stop.

The next day it was Nick's and Mom's turn to see me bald. Both of them were great about it. They may have had some sadness, but neither one showed it. They didn't have any questions either, but Mom did ask me how I felt about it. I reminded her of what I had been saying all along while I was buying wigs, "My hair better fall out or I'll be pissed off." Now all my family had seen me bald and everyone was fine about it. Of course all my body hair eventually fell out. I was very happy about that too. No more need to shave!

With this cycle, my side effects started a day earlier, and as before, the chemo haze was the first to arrive. Only a few hours later I could feel the body pain. That evening as Randal and I relaxed in the living room I began to get extremely fatigued. By now I was very sick. I remained in the living room watching one of my favorite programs while I kept fighting the yawns, and laboured to keep my eyes open. At 8:30 pm I surrendered to my side effects. Not much sense battling something I was going to lose. I took my evening cocktail of drugs, attended to mother nature and slowly climbed my staircase. Once I was in my bedroom I didn't have enough strength to put on my pjs, so I climbed in my bed completely naked. Who cares! I always used to sleep naked, but since the mastectomy I am no longer able to do it, unless I'm too sick and exhausted to care. Asleep by 8:35 pm.

I had a beautiful night's sleep. I didn't wake up until 9:00 am. I was very sick. The first side effect to welcome me to the day was heartburn. It was severe. It felt like I had a bowling ball sitting on my neck and chest and the burning was intensely painful. Immediately I got up to go downstairs to drink some antacid. This day was the first time I could not make it to the toilet on time. As I hurried down the stairs the pee hurried down my legs. I was angry by this. The pain in my feet made my journey downstairs even more horrible. Finally I made it to the bathroom and was able to finish properly on the throne. I then drank the antacid and some water. I found the water helped more than the liquid antacid and the pills. I then took my morning meds and went back upstairs to put on the housecoat I now called "Old Reliable". I ventured downstairs again and plunked myself down on the couch. I decided it was a good time to inject myself with the Neupogen before I showered. I realized this morning I would be very sick for the next two weeks.

During these two weeks while I was very sick, all I could really do was lie in bed and think. I thought about many things. Cancer changes a person, and some of my beliefs and priorities were changing rapidly. Cancer continued to teach me what is important and what is not important. Cancer mellowed me in some ways, and fired me up in other ways. I no longer made a big deal about certain things I used to believe were important, and was becoming more tolerant of others. I started to understand other people better and was becoming less self centered. I came to believe (truly believe, not just think) people are to enjoy what they have, and to strive for more is a good thing. I don't just mean material items, I mean family, home, relationships, friends, faith and enriching the lives of others. People (including myself), should enrich the lives of others through love, kindness, and patience. One should appreciate what and who is around them and relish in it - cherish such gifts, because they could be lost at any time. Once I had good health, but took it for granted - now it was gone. I promised myself to cherish all I have in life and never forget it can be lost in a snap! Once I worried about everything, but now I really had something serious to worry about. I believe worrying helped make me sick to begin with, and that could have killed me. ***"Who of you by worrying can add a single hour to his life?" (Matthew 6:27)*** I was changing in another major way.

My emotions were becoming less and less predictable. There would be days when everyone was at work and school and I would cry all day. At times I would feel normal (as close as normal can get while on chemo), and then suddenly I would become profoundly sad. I remember one day in particular I started to cry, because Randal did not buy my favourite cereal, "God, how thoughtless. He can't even make sure I have my favourite cereal?!" All the other thoughtful acts of kindness he showed me didn't matter at that point. His failure to keep me well supplied with my favourite cereal out shadowed everything else.

Sometimes I would dwell on stupid things I had done in my past and cry about them. I would think about a time when I hurt another person and cry about that. I would recall childhood memories and cry because my childhood was over. I would remember the joy of my childhood and wish I could be five years old again happily playing with my Barbies and baby dolls. I would recall my adolescence and cry about the good times and the not so good times. One morning I stood at the French doors in my bedroom and saw something so sweet and simple it caused me to watch while the tears flowed down my cheeks.

I saw a young couple walking hand in hand down my street. As the tears welled up in my eyes I thought, "What a beautiful sight." Like most people I have seen this sight a hundred times before, but never saw the simple beauty of it. Being very moved by this couple, I was reminded of the days past when I was young and in love with a boy. Those were wonderful days, but oh so fleeting! I envied the couple for their youth. I thought this couple most likely believed their sense of euphoria would never come to an end. That is what I thought at that young age. Their health and their freedom made me want to jump out of my skin and go back to a better time. I wanted to shout out to them, "Be happy! Hold on to what you have now because it won't last forever!" Imagine a bald woman in a light green housecoat shouting to people to be happy. They would have thought I was out of my mind, and if I was one of them I would think the same thing. I watched them turn a corner and could no longer see them. I finished crying and set about my day, but moments like this would happen again.

Days before my next cycle I heard Randal come home from work for lunch. He made the usual sounds in the kitchen and I made no attempt to even move, much less go downstairs and welcome him home. Minutes later I heard him climb the staircase and enter our room, "Hello." he greeted me and I returned with a flat, "Hi." He walked over to me and handed me a piece of Havarti, my favourite cheese, "Here, eat this. I don't think you are taking care of yourself." I was too weak and "zoned out" to explain I didn't have the energy to take care of myself, but I took his offering and really enjoyed it. "Why don't you come downstairs and I'll make you something to eat?" When he left the room my mind suddenly came back from "zoning out" and I made my way to the kitchen where Randal and I enjoyed our lunch together.

One evening, my good friend Joanna phoned me. She had to go to Edmonton to write an English exam and would be there for a few days. She wanted to know if I would come along. She asked the right woman at the right time; I jumped at the opportunity. Being away from home, away from daily reminders of my illness and shopping at the West Edmonton Mall with a close friend was something I wasn't about to pass on. I was still feeling sick, but the trip was falling on the tail end of my third cycle. I believed I would be healthy enough by that time to go. Joanna and I were really looking forward to our escape.

What an escape it was! Filled with enthusiasm and excitement, Joanna picked me up at 8 am and off we went. We had decided not to stay at the hotel in the mall. Although beautiful, the rooms are very pricey, and we wanted to spend our money on other things. When we arrived in Edmonton at 7 pm I suggested a motel my family and I stayed at a couple years prior. It was not a fancy establishment, but it was clean and reasonably priced. We pulled in at the office and soon had our keys. The manager was a friendly man and gave Joanna directions to the university as her exam was early the next morning. Once at our room Joanna asked me to look the room over quickly while she began to get the luggage out of her trunk. My cursory look was over very quickly, and nothing appeared to be wrong with the room. I walked down the stairs to help Joanna with our bags and told her the room appeared fine.

However, it was not! After we had our bags in the room Joanna took a look around herself. She began in the bathroom, when I heard her gasp. She came out and exclaimed, "There are black hairs in the bathtub." Immediately I went and looked and sure enough when I looked closer I could see the hairs. The hairs were encrusted in a layer of scum. Yuck! The toilet and sink were not much better. Minutes later Joanna gasped again, "The police are outside." I looked out the window and yes, two police cars were outside our window. I looked around the exterior of the building from our window and noticed the clientele that was outside. They were less than desirable. We closed our drapes and I went to lock the door. I turned the door knob, locking it, but I couldn't believe what I saw. Usually motels and hotels have a deadbolt as a secondary precaution, but this motel had one of those cheap chains. Both of us were tired and shocked, and decided to leave to get something to eat. During our supper we decided to stay the night, but get a different room the next night. We returned to our room and things just got worse.

Once back in our room Joanna put the cheap chain across the door and we both hoped for the best. I felt so responsible about our room. It had only been two years since my family and I stayed there, and it was acceptable then. There had even been other families staying there. Joanna inspected her bed and found more hairs, both on her sheets and pillow. Right away I inspected my bed and pillow and didn't find anything. I suggested to Joanna she share my bed, and she would have, if it were not for the male ejaculate on her side of the headboard! Again Joanna gasped, "Look at your headboard!" I looked and gasped, "Oh my God! Oh that's gross!" We could not believe what we saw. It's one thing to find some hairs, and quite another to find a strange man's DNA. I walked over to the window and peaked outside. I saw numerous men hanging around and parties going on in other rooms. Then I noticed something that made all this make sense. I saw a harsh younger looking woman walking towards a room with an older man about one foot behind her. She unlocked the door and they both went in. I immediately turned to Joanna and told her what I saw. We were staying at a brothel disguised as a motel!

We really didn't know what to do, both of us so tired and Joanna had to get up early the next morning for her exam. Then we heard the people next door. They were playing terrible loud music and it was obvious they were having a party. We noticed there was no deadbolt on the adjacent door either. We were nervous now, so we stuck one of the cheap chairs at the dining set under the doorknob. We understood this motel was full of prostitutes, druggies, drug dealers and most likely some were in possession of weapons. Neither Joanna or I had anything we could use as a weapon. A chair under a door knob and a cheap chain was all we had to secure ourselves. It was getting late and we both dreaded having to go to bed. Understandably, Joanna refused to share my bed, so she decided to sleep on top of her bed. I had brought a blanket from home and offered it to Joanna. As I passed it to her I said, "Don't worry about my blanket. The only thing on it is pussy hair." She knew I meant my three cats and we shared a much needed laugh. Joanna graciously accepted my offer and we decided it was time to get some sleep.

We didn't get too much sleep that night. We were relieved there was not much noise from the room next door despite the party. I woke up at 6 am and lay in bed hoping I could fall back to sleep, but had no luck. I looked out the window and it was a beautiful, sunny June morning. I opened the door to enjoy the fresh air, and was careful not to wake Joanna. I sat down on a chair in the doorway and noticed a man on the other side of the balcony. I didn't pay much attention to him until he started walking towards me. Before I could close the door he approached me and asked, "Do you have a time?" I told him it was 6:00 am. Not satisfied with my answer he again asked, "No, I mean do you have a time?" Realizing what he meant I bluntly stated, "The only time I have is 6:00 am." and I quickly shut the door and put the cheap chain across door. Joanna woke up and asked what had happened. I explained the story and exclaimed, "How desperate is he? I'm bald. I look like a cancer patient, I'm wearing an old lady housecoat, and it is 6:00 in the morning!" Men never fail to astonish me!

Joanna and I both passed on having a shower, and she quickly got ready to leave for the university. She phoned for a taxi and when she revealed her location the man on the other end of the phone asked, "Are you sure that is the correct address?" I guess this motel is well known in Edmonton for its clientele. After Joanna left I got myself ready to go to the West Edmonton Mall. Joanna left me her car, so I could drive there, and we knew we were not going to return to this motel - ever!

I was proud of myself for being able to drive to the mall without getting lost. I felt somewhat lonely and missed Joanna's company. I had hours to shop by myself, and I really wanted to buy another wig. I was so relieved when I found a wig store within minutes of walking into the mall. I found the wig I wanted the second I entered the store. I have always been attracted to the fashion of the 60's and I found a wig straight from that decade - the popular inverted bob, and it was a beautiful blonde color. An Asian family worked at the store and when I pointed to the wig I noticed the mother take a wig from a drawer. Their English was very poor, so I went to the chair in front of the mirror for a fitting. I pulled off my wig, exposing my bald head and instantly their attitudes towards me changed. They became very kind and helpful, giving me a generous discount when I paid for the wig. My eyes filled up with tears as I handed the cash to the mother and they could see a tear roll down my cheek. I thanked them and the father told me to take care of myself. What kind people.

The kindness of this family touched my heart. God gives us His people. He gives us what we need even when we don't realize we need it. I thanked God for giving me the gift of the kindness of strangers and allowing me to find the wig I really wanted. As I walked away from that store I walked with a lighter step and felt good about myself. A man about 40 years of age was approaching me and he gave me a certain kind of smile. He was a handsome man and I was surprised he looked at me "that way". I almost said, "I won't tell if you don't tell." I felt even better about myself now. Not much later, while I was walking, a woman came out of a hair salon and said to me, "I love your hair. You walked by my salon twice and your hair caught my eye. It looks really sharp." I thanked her as my self esteem began to rise. She continued, "Seriously, your hair looks great." Wow! I sure needed that. I felt great about myself the rest of the day. *"A word aptly spoken is like apples of gold in settings of silver." (Proverbs 25:11)*

I wished my body felt as great as my attitude. My body pain was still an issue and as the hours passed the pain worsened. The fatigue was also getting worse. In the afternoon I went to Joanna's car and took a nap in the backseat. I rested for two hours before I had to meet Joanna at a pre-arranged location. I sat down in front of the department store and my body was completely exhausted and sore, especially my feet. I waited and waited and no Joanna. I began to worry about her after she was one hour late. When we finally met, she explained her tardiness was the fault of the bus system and complimented me on my new wig. She was ready to do some shopping, and I didn't dare tell her how exhausted and sore I felt. I kept my mouth shut as she shopped as much as she wanted. She still does not know just how exhausted I was that evening.

Joanna and I went to the Olive Garden that night for supper, and both of us really enjoyed our meals! Afterward, we attempted to find Ikea. The night before when we got our room at the brothel, the manager gave us directions to get there. We had attempted to find Ikea before settling down at the brothel, but we got lost. We asked the waiter at the restaurant for directions and we made another attempt. We got lost again. We decided to find a nice hotel, which we did. We both had a shower and spent the rest of the evening watching murder mysteries on T.V.. We each had our own hair and ejaculate-free beds and slept beautifully. The next morning we went back to the mall and shopped for a few more hours. We left the mall and tried to find Ikea again, and I am embarrassed to admit we got lost again. Guess it wasn't meant to be. That was when we decided it was time to begin our trip back home.

Our drive back home was just as enjoyable as the trip there. We talked non-stop, and I felt fortunate and thankful to have such an awesome friend. Joanna moved to Canada from Poland after meeting the man of her dreams. It's just too bad he turned out to be a Canadian wart-infested frog. Joanna worked at the care home when I started there. It was her first job after leaving the frog. I could easily sense she had suffered her share of hardships in her marriage. She was like a wounded sparrow/very delicate. She was experiencing her share of job related stress. This angered me and I took it upon myself to do whatever I could to help her with it. I know what it is like to live in a foreign country and it is definitely not easy. I was not about to allow my fellow Canadians to take advantage of this woman just because it was easy. Joanna eventually worked out her issues with the job and everything turned out well. Yes, I am very lucky to have such a great friend! This trip to Edmonton with Joanna is one of my most memorable and special experiences of my life.

As much fun as I had with Joanna, it felt great to get back home. I was exhausted and my entire body ached and ached. Randal greeted me back and I told him all about the experiences Joanna and I had. He was very surprised about the brothel. He filled me in on everything that happened while I was gone. I showed him all my purchases before allowing my exhaustion to defeat me. I spent the evening in Old Reliable and went to bed early. I did not feel any better the next morning, and I was deeply depressed when I woke up.

When I came downstairs Randal was in the living room, and he greeted me with a warm, "Good morning." I was depressed and bitchy, and returned his warm hello with a curt, "Morning." This morning I hated him! I was puzzled by my emotions and knew I was about to have a rough day. I joined Randal in the living room, and he tried to make conversation with me by asking, "How do you feel this morning?" I didn't want to tell him how depressed I felt, so I gave him a quick reply, "Shitty." He could clearly see I was in a very bad mood, and asked, "What's wrong?" I hate when he asks me this question, so I replied with the classic response women usually give when something is wrong, "Nothing." Randal did not press the issue. I continued to remain in the living room and as I sat there I thought negative thoughts about him. This made me feel even more depressed. I couldn't stand to be in the same room with the monster, so I decided to return to my room - and the crying began.

I laid on my bed and cried uncontrollably. I thought about all the sad things that have happened in my life, and dwelled on all the things I should have done in my life. Such self-defeating behaviour! I looked in my cedar chest at all the keepsakes from my kids childhood and wished I could go back in time and relive those happy times. I was feeling sorry for myself, and didn't care. I was depressed about everything. My heartburn was terrible, so I went downstairs to drink some water and antacid. As I walked through the living room the beast I married didn't say a word to me and I quickly returned to my den of woe and resumed the crying. Later in the afternoon I came downstairs to get something to eat. Randal had heard all the crying and he looked at me and asked, "Are you going to be okay?" I replied with a weary, "Ya." After returning to my room once again I dwelled on all Randal's negative traits and all the times I felt hurt by him. I was wallowing in self pity. As afternoon became evening my crying and sense of despair lessened, and instead of dwelling on the negativity regarding Randal, I remembered the goodness and kindness Randal has bestowed upon me.

My fourth cycle was only days away and I still didn't feel any better.

Cycle Four

When I arrived at the hospital I did not feel much better. However, I was happy, because this was my last cycle of the red stuff. Virginia was away on holidays and I was the only patient in at that time. It was nice to have Janice all to myself. As Janice went about her business administering to me, we enjoyed a great conversation. We shared a lot of personal stories about ourselves and I learned a lot about Janice. I told her how excited I was about Matthew's upcoming high school graduation, and I also told her how happy I was to be finished with the red stuff and the Neupogen. I was looking forward to feeling better.

The day after cycle four had me feeling as sick as I was before the chemo treatment. I was so disappointed that I did not feel good between my cycles. I was too fatigued to do any housework, and Mom had the flu, so she could not come over and help. I was stuck in the misery of chemotherapy. Rather than improving, my side effects worsened because I was still sick from my third cycle. I felt that horrible chemo haze and hoped it would not last long. The heartburn was much more worse, and I was desperate for relief. The body pain and the fatigue were considerably worse, as was the pain in my feet. My emotions were fair, but I was becoming depressed. Previously, I had days of depression, but now depression was more frequent and lasting longer.

One morning started out terribly. After everyone left the house I lay in bed feeling the worst that chemotherapy has to offer. I felt like disappearing from the face of the earth, the depression was so intense. I prayed for God's given rest from the pain and for help with the deep depression I felt. I got my pain filled fatigued body out of bed and made my way downstairs to go to the bathroom. I drank some antacid and water, and took my morning meds. My feet ached all the way as I climbed the staircase back up to my bedroom. I opened my French doors and stepped out on the deck. I listened to all the different sounds and the aromas of summer were sweet. That was the first time I realized I was no longer a part of the world. Cancer had isolated me from the world I could see before me. I noticed a man walking down the street, and I wished that could be me. I wondered if that man knew how lucky he was to be able to go for a walk. I cried as I missed being a part of the world around me and saddened by the thought of another day of pain and sickness. I cried as I stood looking at my neighborhood from above knowing I was no longer a part of it the way I once was. I prayed for God's strength, and couldn't imagine how I was going to get through this day.

There wasn't anything to do in my room, so I slowly trudged my way downstairs and completed my morning rituals. I stood in the living room and could not bring myself to watch T.V., but what else could I do when feeling so sick and fatigued? I decided to watch "The Passion of the Christ". I put the movie in the DVD player, and watched about 20 minutes of it. I then decided to go back up to my room, get out of Old Reliable and get dressed in my "kicking around" clothes. As I entered my bedroom I could see the clouds outside my French doors. All my life I have enjoyed looking at clouds, so I walked up to the window to get a better look. I could not believe what I saw!

There before me was the image of an older man sitting on a big chair - a throne! He wore a robe and was entirely majestic with a lion resting at his feet. This image was so clear and detailed. I immediately fell to my knees and prayed as the tears flowed uncontrollably. It is my belief God gave me an image of Himself in the clouds to comfort me on this depressing morning. While I marvelled at the image, I noticed another image below it. I saw an image of a lion with a lamb sleeping beside it. I was amazed. All I could do was rest on my knees as I praised God for this gift. As I was marvelling at the sights, I noticed the cloud formation above the lion and lamb appeared to be a head and profile of the face of a younger man. This man had short curly dark hair with dark features, and I believed it to be Jesus. He was embracing and protecting the lion and the lamb. I stepped out on my deck to look at the images. All of them were so distinct, and again I could not believe what I was seeing. Above this image was a third cloud formation in the image of a large cat. When I looked at it the cat turned its head to me and appeared to be looking at me. I believed this was God's way of reassuring me that my cherished Shin was with God.

We found Shin when he was a tiny kitten in Korea. His mother abandoned him and from our apartment we could hear his distressed kitten calls. Matthew and I went and found him. He was orange and white and very frightened. We took him back up to our apartment and he became an important member of the family. We named him Shin because it meant "new" in Korean. Shin also means "shoes" in Korean, so sometimes I would call him "New Shoes", or "Shin Shin". Oh, how I loved that cat! When we returned to Canada, Shin came along. One summer night a few years ago, Shin was run over by a truck in front of our house. I was heart-broken! I was so angry at God for allowing Shin to die, especially the way he did. I prayed often that God would let our cherished pets live on after death. I prayed Shin would once again be mine someday, someplace, and here this cat in the sky looked down at me! I still feel the pain of losing Shin, but I do believe he will be my pet again. I love and miss you, Shin!

There was yet another image to look at. I noticed between my two big trees there were two angels. They were child-like, and were side by side. I could only see their heads. One was turned towards the other as if telling a secret to the other. They had beautiful curly hair with flowers adorning them. It was a very beautiful image and I stared at it for a long time. There was a third angel between the cat and the older man on a throne. This angel had no wings, but was clothed in a long robe with long hair. This image was not as clear as the others.

Many people look at clouds and try to see something in them, but this was different. I did not have to try to see an image. The image was already there. It was as though God had painted me a picture in the sky and all I had to do was look at it. I continued to look at all the images and was astounded by how long they lasted. Clouds move quickly, but these remained still for a significant amount of time. As I stared at the clouds, I cried and thanked God for His great gift of encouragement. I stared until the clouds shifted into unrecognizable formations. I felt disappointment when it was all over, but felt encouraged, comforted and honoured God helped me in the manner He did. That was one of the most special gifts God has ever given me! I was able to get through the day with a positive attitude. I didn't tell anyone about my experience, but every time I thought about it I smiled. I felt this experience was private - between God and me.

Randal came home that day with the same nasty flu my mom had. I wouldn't let him anywhere near me, fearing I would catch it. We took turns with our bed and I made sure we did not share any pillows and blankets. Once Randal returned to work, Mom was finally able to come over. She hadn't seen me in a month, and was shocked by my appearance. She did not realize how sick looking I had become in a month. She kept staring at me and when I politely asked her to stop she said, "You look like a cancer patient." I agreed. My bald head was accompanied by gray skin, sunken eyes with very dark circles. Everytime I looked in the mirror I felt terrible about myself. I wondered if I would ever look like myself again. My appearance was very depressing to me.

One afternoon I was feeling depressed about everything and didn't know what I should do about it. I felt helpless. I did not want to phone my mom and talk to her about it as I knew this would cause her to worry about me. I decided to phone Lydia. As soon as I heard her voice a lump grew in my throat, and as soon as she said, "How are you doing?" I exclaimed, "Oh Lydia, I'm so depressed!" She wondered why the anti-depressants were not working, and I explained they do work. If I wasn't on anything, my depression would be considerably worse. Lydia helped me sort out my emotions and we even shared a few good laughs. At this point all I could hope for was an easing of my depression and side effects before Matthew's graduation ceremony.

Two of my side effects were getting worse and proving to be quite bothersome. The first side effect to worsen was incontinence. Due to the amount of water I drank my bladder seemed to be pushed to the limit at times. As soon as I felt the urge to urinate I immediately went to the bathroom, but during the night it was more challenging. I would have to get up frequently and many times the urine would trickle down my legs as I hurried to the bathroom. Being late to the tiolet was an everyday occurence in the mornings, and I just hated this. Despite my feelings I had to accept it as part of my illness and treatment and remind myself that it would pass.

The second side effect to become much worse was "chemo brain". The short term memory loss bothered not just me, but everyone around me. Sometimes I would forget important things and inconvience others. This always made me feel terrible and not everybody was understanding about it all the time. Sometimes I would go to say something to someone and the second I opened my mouth I had forgotten what I wanted to say. Sometimes I would walk into a room for something and once there forgot what it was that I wanted. Once when I went to the doctor I had forgotten half of what I needed to tell him. That was when I had to start writing lists. The memory loss was very frustrating and at times I thought I might be losing my mind. I prayed often for God to help me keep it together, especially with the graduation approaching.

Matthew's father and stepmother were driving up from Vancouver Island for the ceremony. They drove up with their two boys for Nick's graduation three years ago, and I really enjoyed their company. After Nick's ceremony we had them all to our house for a barbeque. We were all very civil with each other, which is rather remarkable given our past history. When I think about all the fights and struggles for power we had in the past, I feel deep regret.

Divorce is one of the worst hardships one could ever experience, and I don't wish it upon anyone. My ex-husband and I should have co-operated more with each other, and we are both to blame for all the negativity after our breakup. I have no problem admitting many of our conflicts were the result of my resentments and immaturity. As with most regrets in life, I wish I could turn back the clock and be the person I should have been. I'm sure my ex-husband has his own regrets, but he should be as proud as I am of our kids. I know he is. The kids are close to their father and their step family and I am truly happy about that.

The days passed and my side effects continued to remain a hard reality of my life. It was now only a matter of a few days before the kids' father and his wife would arrive in town. At this point I realized I would not recover from my fourth cycle in time for Matt's graduation. I was so fatigued and I knew the graduation would take every bit of strength I could muster up. In addition to the graduation ceremony the school held another ceremony called, "The Grand March". This was an opportunity for each graduate to perform a formal march and dance with the parent of the opposite sex. Nick had declined to participate in this, but I knew Matt would choose to be a part of it. I knew this day would be long and difficult to get through, but I wanted so desperately to make it the best I could for my son.

The kids' dad arrived on time a couple days before the graduation. They drove up with their fifth wheel and camped in one of the local campsites. The kids spent all their time with their dad while he was in town. I thought that was completely appropriate and I harboured no ill feelings because of it. I didn't do anything but remain in Old Reliable, conserving as much energy as I could for Matt's big day.

Finally graduation day arrived. I had bought a new dress, and because I was experiencing hot flashes and waves of the chills, I took a sweater with me. I wore my favorite blonde wig and applied my make up happily, but I was so very exhausted with each movement. While Matt went to the high school, Nick and Melissa went to the ceremony with their dad. Mom, Randal and I arrived at the high school late and had a difficult time getting a seat. Oh, was I fatigued! As we searched for a seat all I wanted to do was lie down where I stood. We found a seat and I felt so relieved to be able to rest. The ceremony was tediously long, and I couldn't wait to leave. Oh, how I wished I wasn't sick and exhausted. When it was over we took pictures and I found the kids dad very standoffish - not like before. I believe it had to do with my illness. The attitude of some people can be surprising when illness strikes.

I found it very important not to judge the attitudes of people during my illness. People deal with these types of situations in their own ways, and I accepted that. I had thought my kids would have been around me much more than they were, but they were not. I believe they found it very difficult to see me as I was. I always kept myself well groomed, and now I looked absolutely horrific! My figure was destroyed by the steriods, my face had become distorted due to puffiness; I was unrecognizable. My mom said the only part of me that was the same was my voice. Chemotherapy is ugly and it shows itself dramatically. My advice to survivors is to do whatever possible to maintain one's self-esteem. It was important to me to look the best I could for Matt's graduation.

After the graduation ceremony, Mom, Randal and I returned home and rested until it was time to go to the Grand March. I was so sick and tired, and couldn't bear the thought of going out in the heat again, but I had to for my son. Matt was late getting to the high school and it was exhausting waiting for him, and for this ceremony to finally begin. Finally the moment arrived for Matt and I to march and I felt so proud to be his mother. I wanted everyone to know this was my son, and I was glad I pushed myself to participate. The Grand March lasted for about an hour, and soon it was time for him to be off with all his friends for their own celebrations. I went home exhausted and couldn't wait to see Old Reliable.

In preparation for my next round of chemo I went to the doctor to get my usual prescriptions. I also noticed I was coming down with a sinus infection and was given an antibiotic. I patiently waited for the pharmacist to complete my prescriptions, and when they were finished I was more than ready to pay and go home. When the friendly cashier pleasantly directed me to come and pay, I noticed a strange expression on her face. She looked like she was about to cry, then she said to me, "There's something I've been wanting to say to you for a long time." I didn't know what this could possibly be, and in a warm and truly caring manner she said, "I'm praying for you." I was so touched by her kindness I began to cry. I could see her concern written all over her face as she asked, "Is it bad?" I knew she meant the chemo and I replied honestly, "It's really bad." She felt bad because of my tears and apologised for making me cry. She handed me a tissue and still shaken I said, "No. It's good. You did good." Once again I was given the gift of the kindness of strangers when I truly needed it. This cashier touched my heart and spirit in a way no one else had, *"…the tongue of the wise brings healing."* (Proverbs 12:18). I will never forget what she did for me that day. Thank you!

My next round of chemo would start the following week.

Another Descent into Chemotherapy

My comfort in my suffering is this, your promise preserves my life.
(Psalm 119:50)

The morning I was to begin my second round of chemo was a beautiful sunny day in July. Still feeling the effects of the previous chemo treatment, I made my way to the hospital. When I entered the hospital I noticed pink ribbons leading to somewhere. I instantly remembered Janice telling me when I returned for my next cycle there would be a new location for the chemo room. I followed the pink ribbons and when I entered the new room, both Janice and Virginia greeted me with their warm smiles. "Wow!" I exclaimed. This room was huge compared to the Breadbox. Their desk was dwarfed in this room, as were the recliners. Instead of two recliners there were three now. The portable wall of charts was replaced with a permanent one. There was a small fridge and a cabinet with a water cooler, coffee, tea, candies and cookies - wonderful. There were extra chairs for others to sit in when waiting on loved ones to receive chemo. This room was far superior to the Breadbox; the only element that remained was the warm welcoming atmosphere.

I was the only patient when I arrived for my injections. I settled myself into a recliner and both nurses asked me how I was feeling. I told them I was still sick from the red stuff. Oh how I hated the red stuff! I asked how long it would take for the effects of this stuff to wear off and was told it shouldn't take too long. Another positive aspect was no more Neupogen to boost my WBC! My second round of chemo would consist of Trastuzmab

(Herceptin) and Palliate (Taxol), and would run slowly (six hours), to ensure I did not have an allergic reaction. I was also given Benedryl as a precaution. Virginia began the process as Janice kept herself busy at the desk. Virginia warned me that the Benedryl would cause drowsiness and I could possibly fall asleep. As the chemo dripped another patient came in for treatment.

This patient was an older woman, and she was friendly and in good spirits. Janice began her therapy as the woman talked and talked and talked. Despite the pleasant nature of this woman I was annoyed by her constant babble. Another nurse entered the room and everyone was talking, annoying me even more. I started to feel odd, forgetting Virginia's warning. I couldn't keep myself level and thought there was something very wrong. At that point Virginia asked me if I was getting drowsy and then I remembered. She gave me a blanket and a pillow while I reclined my chair. I lay there drifting off to sleep while everyone else talked. In no time lunch arrived and I fell back asleep when finished. The other patient was already gone when I woke up, and soon I was able to go home. I was exhausted and went to bed as soon as I got home.

It only took a day to feel the effects of this new chemo. I did not experience that dreaded chemo haze, or the heartburn, but the body aches were severe. It was in the afternoon when I started to feel sick and I lay in Randal's recliner as my body ached the day away. By the weekend I was in bad shape. I had to take Percacets for the pain, but that only worked for a couple of hours. I should have waited two hours before taking more, but I only waited one hour as I could not stand the pain anymore. Sunday was the worst day.

When I came downstairs, Randal was in his chair watching television. I went about my morning routine, and when I saw my reflection in the bathroom mirror I almost fainted. In all my life I had never looked that bad! My skin was grayer than ever and my sunken eyes with the dark circles looked worse than ever. I was extremely weak and had a difficult time walking. I entered the living room and when Randal looked at me I could see the surprise on his face. I was exceptionally sick that day, my emotions were unstable, and I felt like being alone. I spent most of the day in my bedroom with Mia caring for me.

As I laid in my bed I felt my body ache and ache. I couldn't do anything but feel the pain and pray, "Oh God it hurts. Please don't let it hurt so much." I lay there for hours before I found a cheesy movie on T.V., and eventually fell asleep. When I woke up I could hear Randal downstairs in the kitchen cooking supper. I was amazed by how long I slept. Soon I could smell supper cooking, so I slowly and carefully made my way downstairs. Although I was exceptionally sick and fatigued, I finished out my day and prayed tomorrow would be better.

I absolutely believe prayer is as essential to cancer treatment as any other mode of treatment. I prayed all the time. I prayed while doing daily activities. I prayed while being around others. I prayed during quiet times. I prayed at the chemo room. I prayed while at the doctor's office. I prayed as often as I could, and my prayers became effortless. Prayer became a second nature to me. God was my daily companion and I spoke to him all day long. During this time His presence was always close. I felt as though I was living within a cocoon of protection and He was always near me to protect and nurture me. *"For He will command His angels concerning you, to guard you in all your ways; they will lift you up in their hands, so that you will not strike your foot against a stone." (Psalm 91:11-12)* I knew I had to enjoy this time with Him as it would not last forever. I knew once I was better the cocoon that protected me would be gone. My relationship with God deepened each day, and God was always near. All the communicating I did with God gave me whatever it was I was needing - peace, hope, rest, joy, love, patience, understanding, knowledge, strength... He continues to be present around me and has sustained me through all the misery and fear breast cancer and chemotherapy has cast upon me.

Tomorrow arrived and I was no better. It was a beautiful August day and I spent the entire day in my room, crying. I could not see any hope and everything about my life seemed bleak. I lay in my bed praying the body aches would go away, *"O Lord heal me, for my bones are in agony," (Psalm 6:2)* and periodically would go downstairs to take some painkillers. I missed Melissa; she was visiting her dad for two weeks on Vancouver Island. Every time I thought about her, my heart ached and all I wanted to do was wrap my arms around her and tell her how much I love her. I wanted her to know how precious she is to me and how lucky I am that she is my child. As I was concentrating on my daughter, suddenly mother nature came calling. I travelled down the stairs as quickly as I could, but mother nature beat me to the punch. Another day of incontinence! After cleaning myself I returned to the comfort of my bed as I was far too weak to do anything else. I felt so relieved being back under my covers and my head cradled by my pillow. I dozed off a few times, but mostly lay there being zoned out. I can't even recall if I was thinking, or what I was thinking. For that period of time everything was blank.

As time passed I slowly began to feel better, but only a few days before my next cycle. It was a beautiful Wednesday morning when I rose to leave for the hospital. Before dressing, I stepped outside on my bedroom deck. The morning sun warmed my body and I delighted in the comfort it gave me. As I stood in the warmth I prayed God would continue to be with me during this second cycle, and ease the suffering the chemo would cause.

Virginia and Janice were busy at work when I arrived at the chemo room. The very talkative lady was already in one of the recliners receiving her chemo. I sat myself down and prepared myself mentally for this treatment. As Virginia began the process on me, Janice and the talkative lady conversed. Soon the chemo was dripping into my system and this time I decided I would join in the conversation with the older lady instead of being such a drag. She introduced herself as Laura. As we talked, I fought as hard as I could to not fall asleep from the Benedryl, but I was overcome by drowsiness and slept before our lunch arrived. We enjoyed a lovely conversation over lunch and before I knew it, it was time to go home. When I came home, I lay in Randal's recliner and waited for the side effects to show up. I did not have to wait long. The body aches kicked in rather quickly, as did the fatigue. I decided to go to bed and did not get up until the next day.

I experienced many more days like this one, and they were very difficult to get through. I had no idea just how hard chemotherapy would be. That is a good thing because had I known I might have chosen not to go through it. Ignorance is bliss! This chemo was supposed to be easier than the previous, but so far it was just as bad. The body pain was a steady aching throughout my entire body, and was only eased by the painkillers for a couple of hours. I was growing concerned by the amount of Percacets I was taking just to take the edge off the pain, but after a few days I no longer cared. I was taking more Ativan for my anxiety as well and didn't care in the least about my pill consumption. I had to do what I had to do!

Pain, depression and anxiety were beginning to get the better of me. My positive attitude and fighting spirit had become engulfed by my negative mind set. My sense of adventure had gone off on an adventure of its own and left me behind. Oh, what to do? How am I going to get through this? Is this ever going to end? I finally hit the bottom of the bottom. My anti-depressants weren't working anymore, and I felt hopeless and helpless. I hated the feeling of being isolated from the rest of the world. The world was out there; just outside my door, and I was a ball of flesh that had become completely useless.

I hated everything! I hated my pyjamas, especially Old Reliable. I dreaded getting phone calls from the people that cared about me. I dreaded the thought of having nothing to do but watch the T.V.. There was never anything worthwhile on anyway. I dreaded the thought of having to get my useless body up and go to the dreaded doctor's office. I hated looking around my house because every room was messy and dusty. No one cared enough to tidy up, and I looked at the mess and knew I didn't have the energy, nor the desire to do it myself.

I began to spend more and more days wallowing in self pity. I remembered past days when I was at my best and came to believe I would never be the same woman I once was. I couldn't stand to look at myself in the mirror, because what I saw made me feel disgusted. I used to have beautiful long blonde hair. I used to have beautiful long dark eyelashes. I used to have a healthy complexion and enjoyed wearing my makeup. I used to have a slim shapely body, but now it was distorted and puffy from the steroids. I used to enjoy getting dressed, but now the only item I could wear was Old Reliable. I was a shell of the woman I once was, and wallowing in self pity was not helping. I knew I had to go to the doctor AGAIN to see about my anti-depressants.

Dr. Thomson increased my dosage and eventually they began to work, but what's more important is how low my spirit sunk. It's normal to become depressed about cancer and chemo, but it's imperative to keep one's head above the misery. I believe if a cancer patient needs to take a day or two to feel sorry for themselves that is okay. Any longer could easily increase and one might get into a rut, which can be very difficult to get out of. A positive attitude and a fighting spirit is so important to maintain when fighting cancer. Without these essential tools the spirit tends to admit defeat and give up. I prayed God would help me to pick myself up and take back my determination to reach the finish line. During these dark hours I prayed and prayed and prayed. God has not failed me yet!

Cycle three came slowly. I had been so accustomed to having chemo every two weeks, and I found the three week cycle hard to take. When I arrived at the hospital for my third cycle, Janice was away on her summer holidays. Virginia was working and to my delight Laura was already there receiving her chemo. Laura was more than just talkative. Laura was a very sweet little lady. She was petite in stature and due to her hair loss she wore a jet black wig that made her even more lovable. I found Laura cute as a button and came to enjoy every single word that rolled off her tongue. She had many stories and I enjoyed hearing every one of them. I could easily see that Virginia enjoyed our little Laura as well.

Laura found something to read while Virginia turned her attention my way. As Virginia took care of me, I glanced over at Laura, and this may sound odd, but I enjoyed looking at her. Her little body looked so small in the large recliner and I giggled inside at how adorable she looked in her black wig. Her hands and feet were both wrapped in ice to prevent the chemo from remaining in her digits. She had to have a stool plus a couple of thick books in order for her small feet to touch the bottom. She was like a little girl in an elderly body. This woman was special - really special, and I looked forward to hearing more of her stories as I received my chemo.

Laura shared her personal experiences about her ex-husband with us. He was truly cruel! As she relayed her bad experiences I felt so angry at him. How could he treat such a sweet lady like that? What the hell is wrong with some men? They abuse their women and then can't figure out why they die lonely old men. Luckily she has a wonderful husband now and he comes into the chemo room periodically to check in on her. As Laura talked our lunch came and I was having a ball. I wanted Laura to be at every chemo appointment I had because she made this time so rich. Thank you God for the gift of Laura! After lunch I couldn't stay awake another minute and dozed on and off.

Virginia gave me a pillow and blanket and I could hear Laura telling Virginia about her prosthesis, "I'm making another one." Making another one? I was so curious as to how Laura could be making another prosthesis. I tried so hard to stay awake, but couldn't. I finally woke up due to my snoring! I felt so embarrassed, but quickly forgot about it when I remembered hearing about Laura's prosthesis. I sat up in my recliner and asked her if she wore a prosthesis. She explained she refused (like me), to buy a prosthesis for $400.00, so she knits hers. I told her I was amazed by this. She said she got the idea from a friend of hers in Ontario. Her friend knits them and even knits a nipple on them and sells them for $99.99. When she told me how much her friend sells them for I was rather angry. Yarn is inexpensive and the amount needed would cost less than a fraction of a ball of yarn. I thought the price was completely unfair. Some people want to help other survivors and some people want to cash in on one's misfortune. I kept my opinion to myself, not wanting to hurt Laura's feelings. Laura promised me she would bring one of her prosthesis to our next appointment. I couldn't wait to see it and having to wait three weeks annoyed me. When Laura's husband arrived I could see he was very concerned about her, and could tell he truly loved her. I felt good about that as this lady deserved to be loved.

The chemo took about two days to affect me. Saturday morning I woke up feeling sick, but still felt good enough to be productive. Randal was on call that day, so he was in and out all day. I felt very fatigued, and basically spent the day on the couch. My condition worsened over the next two weeks. During these two weeks on the couch every now and then I heard a voice telling me to "write a book." I had heard this same voice tell me to write a book ever since the first cycle of this round of chemo. I kept ignoring it, thinking it was ridiculous - write a book! I kept hearing this command and finally one evening I said out loud, "Okay, I'll write a book." I immediately got up and found some extra packages of school paper, found myself a comfortable pen and in the privacy of my bedroom began to write a book.

Immediately I was having fun! When I was 13 years old on summer holidays I became so bored and relentlessly bugged my mom, "What can I do?" Out of frustration and irritation she tiredly said, "Oh go write a book." and so I did. It was a love story born out of the mind of a young girl. I had so much fun and to my mom's complete relief finally had something to do. I even made a cover for my little book. I drew a young boy and girl sitting under a tree embracing each other. I called my book, "Walk Alone". My mom was so proud of me she showed my aunt and uncle my book. They asked me for permission to read it. A few days later my uncle came over and returned my book and complimented me on it, saying it was a very well written book - a well written book for a 13 girl. My uncle told me he was impressed by my ambition. Of course I felt wonderful receiving such good reviews and from that day on I was in love with writing. Its no surprise my Bachelor of Arts Degree is complete with a major in English and Literature.

My writing became my escape from cancer and chemotherapy. I couldn't wait to be alone to write. I had told everyone I had started a journal, because I didn't want anyone to know I had heard a voice telling me to write a book. I finally had something to look forward to every day. I bought myself pens that felt good to write with and some pretty pink paper with flowers and butterflies to mark each chapter. I wasn't finished with chemo yet and when it got in the way of my writing I used that time to reflect and concentrate on what I wanted to write and how to incorporate my faith within it. Suddenly my breast cancer had meaning! I had a new lease on life! Most of my depression was gone, but not all of it.

I had become very depressed before my fourth and final cycle. I spent most of my time crying when I was alone. I cried when I woke up and cried throughout the day not letting anyone else know about it. My last cycle was approaching and I felt overwhelmed that I would have another four weeks of being sick before I recovered from chemotherapy. I felt like I was at the end of my rope, and wondered how I would be able to get through the next month. My family couldn't help noticing I was depressed. So much for keeping it a secret! I tried as hard as I could not to cry in front of them, but my feelings of helplessness consumed me and I had to cry whenever I felt like it. There is no shame in that. It is important to feel every emotion and let the floodgates open to release the stress of depression and helplessness.

One morning when I woke up Randal was across the hallway on the computer. I felt tremendous sadness and began to cry. I tried to cry quietly, but Randal heard me anyway. He came into our room and held me as I cried. He reminded me of how close to the end I was and I just had to hang in there a little longer. I know he meant well, but I thought to myself, "You don't know how hard this is. Hang in there a little longer! A little longer seems like months! I don't have any other choice. I have to hang in there a little longer." Despite my negative feelings, Randal's attempt at comforting me did work. He reminded me that one day all this would be behind us, but I could not envision it. I was thankful I had Randal to care for me. He was my caregiver above all others and when he wasn't around I had my little Mia.

One evening only a few days before my fourth cycle I was in my bedroom feeling depressed about the coming weeks. It was the beginning of September when I would have my last chemo, and I was grieving the end of summer. Anyone from northern Canada can relate to that! I heard the phone ring and I hoped it would not be for me. The last thing I wanted to do was talk to someone, but Randal called out, "Wendy, Joanna's on the phone!" Why did he have to yell it out to me? I didn't even have the opportunity to whisper, "If it's for me I'm sleeping." I wiped my eyes, cleared my throat and took the call. Joanna began by asking me how I was feeling and then we talked about her job. We always talked about her job because I knew exactly what she was going through, having once worked there myself. Later in our conversation I told Joanna I was feeling sick and how my treatment seemed endless. Then Joanna said something that instantly changed my attitude, "Yes Wendy, but in a few days your chemo is finished. That is all you have left and you're done." I was dwelling on the next three weeks of feeling sick instead of looking at the bright side. Yes, my chemo would be done in a few days! "You're done next week and then that's it." "Wow!" I exclaimed, "you're right! I'm finished next week!" That realization snapped me right out of my depression, and I felt genuinely happy - really happy. After my phone call I went downstairs and told Randal, "Next week I'm done my chemo. Joanna explained it to me." Randal replied with, "Ya, but you still have three weeks of being sick." "I know, but I feel I can get through it knowing that my chemo is finished next week!" My positive attitude was back! The depression was gone! Happiness set in and life seemed good again.

That evening I went back to my writing again and I was reading my women's devotional Bible. I came across a teaching that transformed my writing and drew me closer to God, deepening our relationship like never before. This devotional suggested to find a quiet place to share time with God, "Imagine! God is looking for worshipers. Will He always have to go to a church to find them, or might there be one or two in an ordinary house, kneeling by a chair?" (Elizabeth Elliot, Meeting God Alone). I knew instantly what I was going to do.

That dreaded staircase I slowly had to climb up and down everyday had a modest space underneath it that we used for storage. The next day when everyone was gone I cleared out all the junk. I put useful items in new locations, and threw out stuff that was no longer useful. I took my white bistro set from my porch outside and put it in my little room. There were two shelves mounted on the wall and I put all my Christian books and Bibles on them. I had some posters in my cedar chest I hung up in my new room. Being a romantic, I had kept the top of the first box of chocolates Randal gave me and hung that up as well. I had an old fashioned parlour lamp I put inside. I added some candles, a stuffed cat, an angel clock, my crucifix, a beautiful vase and some family pictures. This was my "God room." Knowing and feeling God's presence around me, I took Isaiah 55:6 as my purpose for my room, ***"Seek the Lord while He may be found, call on Him while He is near."***

I was so excited and proud about my new room, I couldn't wait to show everybody. To my dismay, nobody was impressed by it as I hoped they would be. The kids thought I was turning into a religious fanatic. Mom and Randal were indifferent, but I didn't care. I didn't transform this room for anyone else, but God and me. I believed I had a wonderful little space to be alone, write, read and spend time with God. It was a great little place to hide away from everyone when I felt like being alone.

The morning of my final chemo cycle arrived and I was elated. As I was getting dressed in the bedroom Randal came in and hugged me. He congratulated me on getting through all the chemo. We were both so happy this was my final cycle. Matthew was taking me to the doctor before chemo, so I could get the last of my prescriptions. He sat in the examination room with me waiting for Dr. Thomson to walk in. Dr. Thomson walked in and he was smiling as usual. I had all my prescription bottles lined up for him and reminded him that this was my last day of chemotherapy. He looked at me and said, "Are you sure this is your last chemo?" "Yes," I said. "Really? Are you sure?" I bounced back with, "I want to know what you know." He broke it to me as gently as he possibly could, "You have 13 more cycles left." I could hardly believe what I heard and I could tell Dr. Thomson felt very uncomfortable telling me, "I hate to be the bearer of bad news, but yes, you have 13 more cycles." I looked at Matthew and he looked as puzzled as I did. With shock and horror in my voice I asked, "Really? How ?" Dr. Thomson reminded me I was to have 17 cycles of Trastuzumab. I had only had four so far. He wrote me the usual prescriptions and I left with my heart sunken in a state of shock.

I dropped off my prescriptions and came home. I retrieved my treatment plan and read it carefully. There in black and white it clearly stated the reality I desperately wanted to be wrong. I had 13 more cycles of Trastuzumab to go. Still hoping there was some sort of mistake, I phoned Janice and asked her about it. She explained it to me just as my treatment plan reflected. That was one of my most shocking moments in my life. I phoned Randal at work and told him, and he was heartbroken for me - shocked too! "How come they didn't tell you?" I explained to him there is no mistake and it was written right in front of me in my treatment plan. The reality had been there the whole time, I just didn't realize it. "Oh my God," Randal said, "You're going to be sick and tired of being sick and tired." Oh God, yes! I wasn't even halfway through my treatment yet!

Matthew drove me to the hospital and I felt detached from the world around me. I grudgingly took my place in one of the recliners feeling defeated. Janice was excellent. She didn't dwell on the misunderstanding and went about her business in her usual warm professional way. Laura was there and she had brought her knitted prosthesis as promised. Thank Heaven that sweet lady was there. Her stories took my mind off the shock of my situation until I started to doze off. I reclined my chair back and thought about, "13 more cycles - 13 more cycles after this one! Fuck!" When I woke up Laura was gone and I spoke briefly to Janice. She told me the next 13 cycles wouldn't be as harsh as the previous ones. I asked her if I would still need to take the Percacets and the Ativan, and she told me most likely not. I thought the bright side of this horror show would be a lessening of side effects. I had to come up with something positive. Cycle four was my sickest. I had all the usual side effects, but for the most part I was mentally zoned out.

One afternoon I sat outside to get some sun. Once again I looked around my neighbourhood. I started to think about the human rat race everyone seems to complain about. I've heard people say the human rat race is useless, but I saw the beauty of it that afternoon. The beauty of being able to drive to a nursery to purchase goods, return and better tend the flowers, the beauty of going to the grocery store, the beauty of going to the bank, the beauty of going to work, the beauty of all that the rat race encompasses. For every car on the road, there is someone doing something I could not presently do. Inside the cars, trucks, trains, and planes there were people doing important things that will influence the lives of others. I have come to believe there are more people doing positive than negative within the rat race. I wanted to be a part of the scenes I was looking at from my deck, but God reminded me to be patient. He reminded me I am out of the race for a time. He reminded me no matter how sick I was, I was to enjoy this time and to take advantage of this time. I decided to quit being so jealous of everyone else around me and to take this time to heal my body and to become closer to God.

One week before my next cycle I noticed I was developing another sinus infection -back to the doctor. I explained my symptoms to him, but he thought it was an allergy and I did not get any antibiotics. A couple days later I noticed a putrid smell in my nose and the mucus was a sickly brownish reddish color. During this time I had a terrible time trying to sleep. The first night I had become very restless, but eventually fell asleep. The second night I was extremely restless. I could not stay in the same position for more than a half a minute. I paced the floors and spent the bulk of the night blowing my nose. I knew for sure at this point I did have a sinus infection and it was severe. When Randal got up for work I told him about my situation and his advice was simple and useless. He told me to have a hot shower, which I did, and did not feel any better. I was angry at him for not taking me seriously.

I phoned my mom as soon as Randal left for work and told her how sick I was. I knew my mom would take me seriously. Matthew drove Mom over to my house and as the morning progressed my condition worsened considerably. I almost fainted four times and this was terrifying to me. What a horrible sensation! My mom wanted me to go to the hospital. I was too stubborn and I refused. I was laying on the couch and I moved my head ever so slightly and I felt myself starting to go under. I screamed out, "Mom!" Oh God was I scared! Mom came running and as she sat down beside me I asked her, "Am I going to die today?" Mom reassured me I wasn't going to die, but more importantly she convinced me to go to the hospital.

I had to be so careful when moving because I was dizzy and afraid of fainting. Once at the hospital, a nurse laid me down in one of the examination rooms. I was still very dizzy, but relieved to be at the hospital. A lab technician came into the room and took some blood while I was waiting for the doctor. It was such a slow process. The doctor finally walked in and told me exactly what I had suspected. I had a very bad sinus infection. He put me on an I.V. with gravol and antibiotics. As I lay there with mom and Matthew waiting I was still very restless. I moved frequently on the bed, doing my best to avoid fainting.

My son Nick showed up at the hospital to see how I was. I was still very sick and still very dizzy and restless. Nick and Matt went to MacDonald's to pick up their lunch and bring it back to the hospital to eat. I was far too sick to eat and still trying to get comfortable. A nurse came in to see how I was doing, and I was happy to tell her the nausea was gone. I mentioned to the nurse my plan to see Janice in the chemo room before leaving the hospital. Not five minutes later Janice was at my bedside concerned about my condition. We had a long talk and I told her all the details. She believed I would be well enough for my chemo treatment the next day. I was given a prescription for antibiotics before leaving the hospital. We had been at the hospital for hours and did not get back home until the early evening.

My sons took my new prescriptions to the drug store for me and took me home so I could get some much needed rest. When they came back to my house, I immediately took my pills and went straight to bed. I was still somewhat uncomfortable and my nose was very sore from all the blowing. Eventually I was able to get comfortable in my bed and was able to watch some T.V.. As I flipped through all the channels I came across a Jann Arden concert. I was so pleased to have found such a worthwhile program - one that could comfort my soul. Each song she sang was a comfort to me physically and mentally. I listened carefully to all the words and reflected on my life. Through her music I became content and thankful about everything and everyone in my life. I wished I could climb through the television set and personally thank Jann Arden for the gift of her music. Thank you Jann Arden!

As the night progressed my restlessness returned, and it was much worse than before. I went downstairs to ask Randal to take me back to the hospital, but he was sleeping on the couch. He had been working so hard lately and didn't get much sleep himself. I really didn't want to disturb him, so I remained in my bedroom the entire night. I moved constantly! I put my body in every imaginable and unimaginable position possible. I was in a state of complete and utter turmoil again. I couldn't even begin to suspect what could be wrong with me. I had suffered from sinus infections for years, but never had one this severe. As I continually moved in my bedroom I watched each hour pass. I couldn't even get comfortable enough to waste time watching the television. I was absolutely beside myself!

Morning finally came, I went downstairs and told Randal about my night. He was not very sympathetic and told me to be patient and wait for the antibiotics to start working. Whatever! Feeling disregarded by my husband I returned to my bedroom, and waited for Randal to leave the house. The second he was out the door I was back on the phone with my mom. My chemo appointment was for 10:00am, but I insisted that Matthew and Mom take me to the hospital immediately. When they came over I was so agitated I couldn't even dress myself. Mom came upstairs to help me dress while Matthew waited downstairs. I was so angry while mom attempted to help me. With great effort I found a pair of socks and hit my bed with them repeatedly while bellowing out loud, "I'm so fucking, fucking mad." I was making such a fuss, Matthew came upstairs to see what all the commotion was all about. With Mom's help we got me dressed and to the hospital by 8:30am.

I boldly walked into the chemo room and as Janice quietly worked at her desk I blurted out, "There is something wrong with me. I have to move constantly. I have been awake for 48 hours moving. I can't stay in one position for more than 30 seconds." As I spoke I was pacing the floor. I completely disregarded the lady that was receiving her chemo. I was completely self absorbed and demanding Janice do something. Janice looked at me and politely suggested I have a seat. I did so, but being so restless I was only able to remain seated for seconds. I was on the move again

Janice was excellent. Virginia was back in Ontario, so Janice was on her own and doing very well. She was calm and again gently requested I sit down in one of the recliners. I threw off my coat and pulled off my wig; and feeling exasperated I plunked my butt down in the recliner. I nervously sat on the edge of the chair as Janice pulled up a seat directly in front of me. With a soothing tone Janice said, "Okay Wendy." She then put her hand on my knee and gently rubbed it as she continued, "Just relax and try to calm down. We're going to find out what's wrong." I did as she asked, however I was still feeling very much agitated. Janice wanted to know all the medications I was taking. I told her all the ones I could remember, but my mind was racing.

Janice went to her computer and was able to retrieve a list of every medication I had taken since April 30, 2008. She asked me to describe all my symptoms. As Janice was investigating, I had to get up and move. I kept pacing the floor as I rubbed my bald head with my hand complaining, "I have this one hair that's hard and poking out all above the fuzz. I blurted, "It has been driving me crazy all night. I can't quit touching it." I wondered if everyone thought I was as crazy as I sounded. About 15 minutes later Janice asked me, "Have you quit taking any of your medications?" "Yes. I quit taking the Oxycodone and the Ativan because I didn't think I would need it while receiving only the Herceptin." Janice looked at me and described what my problem was, "Wendy, what I think we have here is drug withdrawals." I'm sure my jaw hit the floor. Janice continued, "You can't go off either one of those drugs suddenly. It's very dangerous. You could have seizures, a stroke, or cardiac arrest. You have to go off these medications slowly." I was so embarrassed I could have crawled under a rock. "Are you serious?" I asked with the humiliation echoing within my voice. Janice was absolutely correct! I was detoxing! She came back over to me and again placed her hand on my knee, "We'll get you fixed up today." Janice left the room and moments later returned with two Ativans. I placed them under my tongue as she said, "If you don't feel any better in 20 minutes I'll give you another one." After twenty minutes she had to give me two more. Janice mercifully cancelled my treatment that morning and scheduled it for the next day. She phoned Dr. Thomson and he said he wanted to see me after I left the hospital.

By the time I arrived at my doctor's office I was high as a kite. The Ativan was working very well. I didn't really hear much of what Dr. Thomson was saying. All I knew was I was getting a prescription for Ativan and Oxycodone (percacet) - thank God! I do remember Dr. Thomson was very understanding and told me as he wrote out the prescription, "Whatever you do, do not go off the Ativan." I felt like a true drug addict and couldn't wait to get those pills in me. Matthew dropped me off at home and later returned with my pills. I anxiously drank them down. I still felt very humiliated and dreaded having to tell Randal what was wrong with me. When Randal came home I had taken enough pills and I felt normal again. I told him the sordid explanation. He was non judgmental and we shared a quiet evening together.

The next day at the hospital Janice was the only person there, much to my relief. I admitted to her how humiliated and ashamed I felt. She assured me I was not a junkie and when the proper time came I would be taken off the pills gradually. Again she explained how much danger I had put myself in and how some people have died from such a situation. She made me feel so much better when she said, "It's not your fault, you didn't know, and we had to get you through that chemo." We even shared a good laugh when she told me what Dr. Thomson said on the phone the previous day, "Oh my God. She's in detox." Janice phoned my doctor after I had left his office the previous day and I laughed when she told me Dr. Thomson said I was feeling very happy when I left his office.

What an experience! I have a lot more empathy and sympathy for others that find themselves in the grip of drug addiction. What an absolute nightmare! I'll never forget how my body felt. Every fibre of my body was screaming out, "I want those drugs NOW!" It is an indescribable feeling, and while feeling it, nothing else matters but getting that drug. It was an experience I will never forget.

Depression

The cords of death entangle me,
The anguish of the grave came
Upon me;
I was overcome by trouble and
Sorrow.
Then I called on the name of the
Lord:
"O Lord, save me!" (Psalm 116:3-4)

While I was in the depths of my treatment I was also in the depths of depression. In order to deal with my depression I had to look at it in a completely untraditional manner. I imagined depression as a legion of demons. In my story Satan gathered his most deceitful demons and named this group "Depression". Satan made it clear to the members of this group to go out into the world, spread out to every corner, and inflict all the misery they carry onto each human being. Satan instructed Depression to be malicious, vicious, relentless, and to concentrate on the main goal: to cause every human being an inner betrayal between the mind and the spirit.

Each demon chose their own subjects and climbed on their backs. From the human back it was easy to reach over to the human ear and begin the work of lying. These demons are heartless and relentless in their work. The subjects were and continued to be young and old, rich and poor, male and female, straight and gay, hungry and full, fat and thin, happy and sad, close to God and far away from God, black and white, and every other color. The only requirement the subjects had was to be human.

Once Depression is successful at causing the mind to lie to the spirit it can begin to be the thief it was intended to be. Depression begins to rob the human of virtually everything - even to the point of life. Depression first steals the human's thoughts and beliefs. It makes it impossible for the human to distinguish reality, so the next element taken by Depression is the human's sense of reality. Depression then progresses to steal all that is important to the human: control, security, happiness, belonging, family, friends, jobs, freedom, peace, love, kindness, sobriety, health….the list is endless. Depression flourishes in barren places and when severe, Depression will cause death on many levels including physical death.

Through my depression I imagined an ugly gray creature resting on my back and whispering his insidious lies. I could feel the misery this creature oozed out and into my mind. I could immediately recognize his lies: You're worthless, you're ugly, you're a loser, no one loves you, no one cares about you, you're going to die, God is a farce, there is no such thing as Heaven, God doesn't love you, You're always bugging God with your endless babble, He's sick of you, God can't hear you, you are God's biggest pest - on and on the devilish Depression lied. When I started to hear these lies I called upon Jesus to deal with the miserable pest as He had done before. ***"What do you want with us, Son of God?…Have you come here to torture us before the appointed time?…The demon begged Jesus, "If you drive us out, send us to the herd of pigs." He said to them, "Go." So they came out and went to the pigs and the whole herd rushed down the steep bank into the lake and died in the water." (Matthew 8:29-32)***

I spoke to God all the time while I was experiencing depression. A survivor must feel the seriousness of cancer and treatment. I truly believe it is important and healthy for survivors to allow themselves a short period of time to wallow in self pity. In my opinion, wallowing in self pity for a time gives us an opportunity to grieve. It is unhealthy to not recognize depression, and unhealthy to ignore the true feelings of sadness. It's okay to feel sympathy for oneself! Cancer and treatment are serious, difficult, and more often than not, depressing. When I allowed myself to feel sorry for myself, it gave me the perfect opportunity to speak to the Father and give Him all my thoughts, feelings and fears. These opportunities drew me closer to God and when it was over I felt a great amount of relief and the depression either eased or disappeared. A strong warning: while wallowing in self pity, it must not linger. If depression and self pity remain it is time to see the doctor and start taking anti depressants. Survivors must not put their health in peril by allowing depression to remain a daily state of mind.

Depression is not a condition any cancer patient can escape. The depression that accompanied me through treatment was different than the depression I suffered before my diagnosis. My depression before cancer was constant. I believed my life was worthless and essentially over. I could not fathom any happiness for myself at any point in my life. I believed my life would become worse as time passed by and that all my future experiences would be negative. The depression I experienced while going through treatment was not constant. It would come in waves and it seemed to come over me for no particular reason. I would be clipping along nicely and then, BAM! I would hit a solid brick wall of profound sadness and depression. I would become depressed about everything, and I mean everything.

The first time depression hit me was in my second cycle of my first round of chemo. I had woken up in the morning feeling great. I was at the tail end of my cycle with the next one just two days away. My mind and body were both healthy. I had a shower, got dressed, put on my make up and styled my hair. It was a beautiful sunny day in May and I had planned to go and sit on my front porch after organizing my living room. As I busied myself, I suddenly began to cry. I stopped what I was doing, sat down on the couch, put my face in my hands, and cried like a baby. "Why?" I wondered. I was astonished by how this sadness engulfed me. I could not stop crying.

About half an hour later the tears finally dried up and I was able to pull myself together. I put on my white hat and my sunglasses and sat at my bistro set on the front porch looking at my neighbourhood. The warmth from the sun comforted my spirit and the peace within my neighbourhood gave me a sense of appreciation for being alive. My sadness was still with me just under the surface. Anything could and did set it off again.

I noticed a young mom pushing her infant child in a stroller. As she approached me the tears that rested under the surface gently rolled down my cheeks. I began to remember the years when I was a young mother and my children were small. When my children were little and underfoot my mom would tell me, "Enjoy them while they're young, because they grow up so fast." Another pearl of wisdom my mom offered me to relieve my exhaustion, "When they're young it seems like they'll never grow up, but before you know it they're grown." How true! My mother's words came to pass after all those years. Children grow up in a blink of an eye. I cried as I wondered where all those years went.

All I ever really wanted in the world was children. Even as a child I dreamed of the day I would become a mom. I was so happy and excited the day I found out I was pregnant for the first time. Despite the nausea and the pre-eclampsia, I loved my pregnant body. Such joy and fascination I would feel every time my baby moved. I marvelled at the way my belly would move as the baby moved within me. I spent months wondering who this little person was inside me, and when Nicholas was born words couldn't begin to describe the happiness and pride I felt. Every mom believes her baby is the most beautiful in the world, but I didn't just believe this. I knew it! I fell instantly in love with my new baby boy. Watching the young mom as she passed by made me realize just how precious those years were and how much I miss them.

I became so upset I had to go back inside the house. Again I cried like a baby. I thanked God for the three wonderful children he blessed me with. I wished I could relive just one of those days. I continued to recall each pregnancy and each birth. As I spoke to God I remembered numerous and precious moments I had once experienced with my children. I did not cry as though my children were grown and gone I cried as though they were dead and buried. Finally I forced myself to quit thinking about the past and think about my kids today as they are in the present.

Hours passed and I was still feeling depressed and still crying about many things. Exhausted, I prayed for peace. Soon peace calmed my spirit and suddenly there were no more tears to cry. The depression left as though it had never come. The thoughts about my children now made me smile. This day was difficult to get through, and I had many more days like this ahead of me.

Feeling the despair depression inflicts is one of the most challenging experiences of the human condition. The addition of a life threatening illness makes this equation deadly. It can not be overstated that depression is capable of cutting a human life short. For the cancer patient it is imperative - absolutely imperative to maintain a positive attitude, and it is absolutely possible to maintain a positive attitude. Survivors must do what they must to fight depression, whether it is imagining depression as a demonic creature to order, "Go", or anti-depressants, meditation, visualization, relaxation, prayer, or exercise. These methods work and they work exceptionally well in combination with each other. Waves of depression are to be expected during cancer treatment. It's okay to allow the wave to flow and run its course. It's okay to allow oneself to feel self-sympathy, and then release it. It's okay and necessary to grieve all the losses cancer and chemotherapy have incurred. It's okay and necessary to surrender to God, loved ones, supporters, and caregivers; and allow them to give rest, comfort, validation, and encouragement.

During my waves of depression I prayed continually, continued to take my anti depressants, and allowed myself to grieve my losses. I allowed the people that love and care about me to help me. Depression is a part of cancer and cancer treatment. Recognizing it is half the battle and steady, proper management will ensure a positive attitude, so necessary for recovery.

The Great Radiation Debate

When I am afraid
I will trust in you.
In God, whose word I praise,
In God I trust; I will not be afraid. (Psalm 56:3-4)

From the very beginning of my journey I knew radiation would not be something I was willing to accept as part of my treatment plan. I can not explain it as something other than God's whispering voice. Long before I got cancer I continually heard the same message from the general health care professionals, especially through the media. The health care profession promotes patients take an active role in their treatment. I interpreted that to mean patients are encouraged to make informed decisions regarding their own treatment. I have heard that some patients completely forgo traditional medical methods and opt for homeopathic remedies. I have also heard of some patients that opt for traditional eastern methods such as acupuncture and other less known treatments. I have heard of some patients whose treatment plan consist of a mere change in diet. Some patients accept all possible treatments. When I attempted to take an active role in my treatment and made an informed decision I had a small battle on my hands.

After my surgery my surgeon told me I would not require radiation, because all the cancer tissue had been removed from my breast and lymph nodes. I was very relieved to hear this, because I had already decided I was not going to allow my body to undergo radiation. Some may call it a gut feeling, but I call it God's guidance. Whatever one wishes to label that feeling, in my experience, that little voice or feeling is usually right. However, I did not want to make such a major decision based on instinct alone, so I did my homework on radiation. I read everything I could get my hands on as well as information from reputable websites, and what I learned did not impress me.

The first negative aspect of radiation was is that it affects breast reconstruction. Is breast reconstruction important to me? Yes! Is breast reconstruction more important than saving my life? No! My decision could not hinge on breast reconstruction alone. Hence, the second negative aspect of radiation - only a 5-8% increase in survival rates among women living 15 years beyond treatment. In my opinion, that is a very modest increase. The third negative aspect was I would have to live at my brother's house in Mission for at least 6 weeks. During this time, he would have to drive me into Vancouver everyday. Finally, being away from my home and my family for such a long period of time would be extremely lonely. In essence I did not have any faith in radiation as a viable part of treatment. I am speaking only for myself! I do not discourage anyone from taking it, but encourage everyone to make their own informed decision about it and all other treatments. During my first four cycles of chemo my mind was made up against radiation, but my doctors had different opinions than me.

I had just finished my first four cycles of chemo when my oncologist phoned to check on me. She asked me when I would be beginning my radiation treatment, and I boldly and confidently told her I had no intentions of taking radiation therapy. She was very surprised by this and wanted to know why I was refusing it. I explained all the negative aspects already mentioned and she became very concerned. She reminded me my cancer was an aggressive one with a high likelihood of recurrence. My oncologist is a caring woman and was greatly concerned by my decision. We continued to discuss the topic. I ended our conversation with a promise to give it more consideration. I hung up the phone and again considered radiation and again decided against it.

The radiation debate came up again after the end of my second round of chemo. My oncologist phoned me again to check on me and took the opportunity to ask me about my decision regarding radiation. I once again boldly and confidently told her I had not changed my mind on the topic, and once again she was very concerned. She did not press the matter too much with me, but when I saw Dr. Thomson later that same day he had something to say about it. I know both doctors were coming from a good place and because I respected their educated opinions, I listened. Dr. Thomson explained all the benefits of radiation and wanted to do everything possible for me, "We are going for a cure and we want to do everything we can, so if you have a recurrence we will at least know we did everything possible. You don't want to look back and wonder if you might have been okay if you had taken the radiation.." I reluctantly agreed to radiation therapy.

I must admit I did feel coerced into doing something I really did not want to do. I did not feel positive about this decision in any way. My family and friends were naturally curious as to why I changed my mind so abruptly. I explained by spouting all the reasons I had been told about the benefits of radiation, "I want to do everything possible to avoid a recurrence." "It is an important part of my treatment plan." "I want to be a part of the 80% of women living beyond 15 years." Blah, blah, blah. The truth of the matter was I was angry.

I was angry for a number of reasons. First, there was now a huge push and rush to get me under the beam as quickly as possible, "because there could still be some cancer cells hiding." I waited two weeks between diagnosis and surgery. Was it safe to leave that 2.5 cm cancerous tumour in my body for two weeks, allowing the cancer cells to thrive and grow some more? I just couldn't wait to have that breast taken off my body, because I knew once it was gone, the cancer would be gone too. After the surgery I had to wait three months to begin chemotherapy. What reason - what good reason for the three month wait? When I phoned to enquire about my much anticipated appointment with the oncologist I was made to feel like a classic pain in the ass. When I returned home in April after seeing the oncologist, I was told my chemo would begin right away. I had waited another two weeks before my first treatment. Suddenly now radiation must not be delayed because it would kill any cancer cells left behind from the surgery and chemo!

The second reason I was angry was simple; my opinion didn't seem to matter to anyone. I was just the cancer patient that needed to ignore everything I have read about radiation and blindly follow the same path the rest of the pack took. That is not me! Why bother to promote patient involvement when clearly it means one should keep one's mouth shut and do as told? Forget making an informed decision and forget trying therapies less known and less trusted. I do not believe the cure for cancer is sitting on a shelf in a health food store. I do not believe there is a great conspiracy between the doctors, researchers, and pharmacuetical companies to keep the public sick in order to make more money. I don't believe every cancer patient is the same, nor should treatment be the same - exactly the same, without deviation or any additions the patient feels is important.

The third reason I was angry was due to the general and pure ignorance of others, who had no clue about cancer and cancer treatment, telling me what I should do. Survival, survival, survival! Yes! From the second I knew I had cancer I wanted to survive. Just weeks prior I wanted to die, but cancer changed everything. I have heard the ignorance of others who have zero experience with cancer. Some people spoke as though they had a shield around them making it impossible for cancer to enter. One person told me they would never get cancer because...! Don't tempt fate! Anyone - anyone can get cancer! Babies and children have new young parts, don't smoke, don't drink, don't do drugs, and live a healthy life, but still get cancer. Healthy people who do everything condusive to the picture of health get cancer, while others drink, smoke, do drugs and live life on the edge for years and don't get cancer. When faced with the ignorance of others, I explained it as follows: Everyone is going to die. No one here gets out alive! Cancer is a crap shoot. It hits some and doesn't hit others. Doctors, children of doctors, researchers and rich people have died from cancer. Advocates of the conspiracy theory sell books and pills that have never been proven to cure cancer. All people around the world are at a risk of developing cancer. Another ignorant comment I heard was from those trying to figure out what caused my cancer. Maybe it was the smoking. Maybe it was the stress of my marriage, family and job. Maybe it was the drinking I did as a teenager. Maybe it was the sun tanning I did as a young woman. Suggestions were endless.

"I am a cancer patient - don't take away my freedom of choice! Cancer has taken everything away from me, my health, my sense of well being, my hope, my ability to earn money, many of my choices, many of my freedoms, my energy, my beauty, my hair....Cancer has changed me and everything around me. To force me to do something I don't want to do is taking away from me the one thing I have left - my choice. For God's sake, let me make a choice like everyone else around me! Okay I was angry, but the essence of me was still somewhere inside, and someday I will be back!"

I travelled to Vancouver in October to see my oncologist and radiologist. Both of my harsh rounds of chemo were behind me and now I only had to complete 13 cycles of Herceptin, begin hormone therapy and begin radiation (maybe radiation). I just hate travelling alone, and knowing Matthew could use a holiday, I made all the arrangements for our trip to Vancouver. My brother Terry and his wife were vacationing in Arizona, but they allowed Matthew and me to stay in their home in Mission while they were away.

It was great having someone with me this time for all my appointments. It was not the circus show I experienced in April. Matthew was with me when I met with my oncologist. Once again she came in and sat down in front of me. This time she looked at me and giggled. I wondered what she could be laughing at that was so funny. Apparently I had my wig on crooked. Another silly moment for a cancer patient. How many times before have I had my wig on crooked in public? More than I care to admit. I laughed too, because what else could I do? Get angry? I had taken such great care to look my best for her, my absolute best, but somehow my wig jiggled its way lopsided. Oh well, small beans compared to what else I had been through in the past months!

Our appointment was very brief. She spoke about the radiation and was very pleased I had agreed to have it. We discussed Tamoxifen. I would be on this medication for five years, but one of the risks of this pill was blood clots. Due to a family history of blood clots I would not be able to take this medication. She had to come up with something different for me. And that was it! Short and sweet.

The following day I met with the radiologist. He examined the breastless left side of my chest. It doesn't matter how many children one has, or how many pap tests one has, or how many breast exams one has, this never gets comfortable. After all the uncomfortable stuff, he explained all about radiation. Matthew was beside me as he described all the risks. He quickly skirted over the fact that women with a history of smoking have a 15% chance of developing lung cancer from the radiation. At that point I stopped him and asked him to repeat what he had just said. Yes, a 15% chance of lung cancer for people with a history of smoking. Smoking, that nasty addiction I took up in high school, believing it made me cool. I instantly changed my mind about having radiation, although I did not say anything at that point fearing I would be coerced into agreeing to it. The radiologist also mentioned any breast reconstruction may be compromised. I already knew that. I knew I would have to weigh the benefits and the risks before making any concrete decision.

Following my Vancouver trip while at my next chemo appointment I read a book about breast cancer in order to pass the time. I immediately turned to the chapter on radiation. I read all the benefits and all the risks. This book also stated the patient must weigh the benefits and the risks and make their own decision. Perfect! That is what I had been trying to do. The reasons I chose not to have radiation are: a compromised result in reconstruction, 15% chance of developing lung cancer, an increase in hardening of the arteries (left sided radiation), hence an increase in heart attack, inflammation of the lungs causing pnemonia. Too risky for me.

I do not discourage or recommend radiation treatment for any other cancer patient. I do however, encourage all cancer patients to do their homework. They know their bodies better than anyone else. All cancer patients know what is important to them and what is not. All cancer patients should seek out the opinions of others, both professional and otherwise, and base any decision on their own health and well-being. As stated previously, this is my cancer, this is my treatment and this is my decision! It's all about me!

Taking my own advice, I asked Virginia that day what her opinion was for me regarding radiation. She did not tell me what to do, but did encourage me to follow my own instincts. Thank you Virginia! Finally someone in the medical field that understood me and the decision I had to make. Three weeks later I asked Janice her opinion about radiation and me, and was delighted to hear she agreed with Virginia - follow my own instincts. Virginia and Janice made me feel like I was the most important person in my treatment. I knew I would not be taking radiation and I no longer cared what anyone else thought about it. That was the end of the Great Radiation Debate.

A True Christmas

Praise Him with the sounding of the trumpet,
Praise Him with the harp and lyre,
Praise Him with tambourine and dancing,
Praise Him with the strings and flute,
Praise Him with the clash of cymbals,
Praise Him with resounding cymbals. (Psalm 150:3-5)

Before my trip to Vancouver in October I had noticed pain and stiffness in my knees. At that time I thought the pain was a side effect of the chemo that would soon disappear. Unfortunately, the pain and stiffness did not disappear, but was becoming more and more painful. By November my pain had become a major issue in my life. Pain and pills can go hand in hand for the cancer patient, and pills were also becoming a major issue in my life. Dr. Thomson and my oncologist could not explain why I had so much pain and why it was worsening. The only explanation my oncologist came up with was chemo-related arthritis. Dr. Thomson prescribed different arthritic medications, all of which failed to work. Dr. Thomson increased my dosage of oxycodone, which did help for some time. I began to feel better and was able to do more around the house. I landed the job at Walmart and was happy to return to the work force, making extra cash for Christmas.

It was November and although I was feeling better physically I was also feeling somewhat down about Christmas. The kids were all flying down to Vancouver Island to spend Christmas with their dad, and I knew

I would feel lonely for them. One afternoon I received a phone call from my sister-in-law, Delphine, that changed my entire outlook. We began our conversation with the usual pleasantries and she then took great pleasure in telling me she and my brother Bryan were flying up to Fort St. John to spend Christmas with us. In fact the plane tickets had already been purchased! I was so happy and excited. This was the best news I had heard in months. I knew this Christmas would be one of my best ever despite the kids absence. Their visit would be my Christmas present! Thanks to Delphine I finally had something to really look forward to. Thank you Deli!

I continued my attempt at working for a living again, but it became more of a challenge than I thought it would be. My pain and stiffness were increasing and so too was the amount of Oxycodone I had to take to control it. Dr. Thomson prescribed Oxycotin three times daily and more Oxycodone for any breakthrough pain. One day at work was particularly bad. I started my shift at 9:00am and only two hours later I felt exhausted. I foolishly forced myself to keep stocking those shelves until I couldn't move another muscle. I went home at noon feeling completely defeated. Cancer won again! I was so very angry. I wanted so terribly to be like everybody else, but I wasn't. I was a cancer patient and I had to accept the limits this disease imposed upon me. I knew I would not be able to keep my job. I had to graciously accept that and graciously carry on with the business of living. I only worked for two weeks.

Shortly after I quit my job friends of ours phoned to invite us to a concert in December. Jann Arden was coming to town and I couldn't be more delighted. I knew I would enjoy her concert in a way most people would not. This woman had unknowingly soothed my anxious spirit while I unknowingly detoxed. This woman would never know me, nor know just how much she helped me one confusing night. I was going to experience her music in person and I couldn't wait until I could feel the wonderful emotions her music provoked in me. I now had another Christmas present - Jann Arden!

On a cold winter's evening in December we travelled with our friends to a nearby city for the concert. I took all my pain and stiffness with me as well as my painkillers and sedatives. I had put on my long brown wig - the one that made me feel young and sexy. I made sure I wore something special to add to my youthful sexy attitude. I took great care applying my make-up, and wore it heavily as well as proudly. I felt great and I wanted to look as good as all the other women - the other healthy women. So many days I had looked as though my death was imminent, but this night I made sure I looked as young and vibrant as possible.

As we waited for the show to begin I thanked God for this gift. God had given me so many gifts since I was diagnosed with cancer, and He gave me these gifts without me even asking for them. How great is that?! I was feeling fantastic. I was out in public with hundreds of people. I was a part of them - a part of the world again. I felt normal! I could exist outside of my house. I could be like other people, like healthy people. As I watched everyone around me I wondered if they knew how lucky they were to be healthy. I concluded most of them were most likely the same as me before my illness - taking their health for granted. "Oh God thank you for letting me be here!" I thought.

The lights turned off. Any moment now Jann Arden would be on the stage and I would hear her beautiful music. Does she realize how important this evening is to me? No, of course not. I'm just another face in the crowd before her. Do performers ever realize the impact they can have on people? Again, I thanked God for letting me be here. The last time I felt this excited about seeing a live performance was back in 1989 when I was lucky enough to see The Rolling Stones. What a night that was! My favourite rock band of all time - The Rolling Stones! Never in my life did I ever think I would be lucky enough to watch them perform in person. Ever since I was a young teenager I loved them, and thought Mick Jagger was absolutely gorgeous. I was seven months pregnant with Matthew as I waited for the Stones to begin their performance. They blasted on stage with "Start Me Up," one of the best songs ever written. I was almost hysterical when I saw them "in real life"! Not believing my own eyes, I actually shouted out to Matt's father, "Look! Look, they're all here! Mick, Keith, Bill, Charlie, Ron! All of them are right here!" I was star-struck. They played all their hits and I danced as Matthew moved continuously in my womb. He liked them too! That was truly one of the best experiences of my life!

This night was too. I was alive! I was alive and lucky enough to see the woman that calmed my soul when I needed it so desperately. Jann Arden and her band came on stage and began to play. Oh God, I am alive and here! How precious to be alive and to listen to music - beautiful music someone created for others to enjoy. I savoured every note she sang. Thank you, Jann Arden, for your beautiful music and the gift you gave me on a cold December night!

The next day it was back to stark reality - pain, stiffness and pills. I had to be a trooper and trudge along as before. When I was first diagnosed with breast cancer I described my illness as a stone I had to kick aside in order to get on with the rest of my life, and that is what I was doing on a daily basis. I was kicking at this stone and slowly it was being forced out of my path. I had to put up with the pain and stiffness that had now invaded almost all my joints. "Oh God what is wrong with me?" I felt depressed about my pain. However, Christmas was fast approaching and I was excited about my brother's arrival.

Bryan and Delphine were to arrive December 23rd. As the day approached I became more and more excited despite my pain and stiffness. Mom and Randal were also excited about their visit. Randal wanted to be the one to pick them up at the airport, but I insisted I would be the one to meet them. He didn't argue with me. After all, I was the cancer patient and it was my family members coming. Mom wanted to come with me to meet them, but there would not be enough room in the truck for everyone, so I arrived at the airport solo. I had left the house a little early that evening and when I got to the airport I found out their plane was delayed by one half hour. I waited anxiously and wondered if they would even recognize me as my appearance had changed so drastically since they last saw me.

Their plane finally landed and I watched as each person walked off the plane into the frigid cold of Fort St. John. Delphine was the first of the two to walk off the plane. I smiled when I saw her wearing her fur coat - sensible attire for northern Canada. She walked into the airport and she recognized me immediately. We gave each other a hug and it felt so good. We watched Bryan walk into the airport and I smiled when I saw him shivering his way inside. My brother gave me a huge hug and again it felt so good. Thank you God for family! I was so happy to have such a wonderful brother and equally happy he and his wife decided to spend Christmas at my home.

Their first evening at my home was spent putting up the Christmas tree and decorating it. I cannot remember the last time we had enjoyed this Christmas tradition together. I felt such a sense of joy during this evening and I know they did too. It was equally joyous spending Christmas day together. I found happiness exchanging gifts with them. I felt a little melancholy about the absence of my children, but I refused to dwell upon it. We all happily pigged out on Christmas dinner together. Later, we relaxed and enjoyed a quiet Christmas night.

It was a great Christmas! A special Christmas. Before cancer entered my life I did not appreciate my family members as I now do. To be with each other is truly precious. Why could I not feel this before as I do now? Oh God, please never let me forget how precious my family is.

My Bout With Drug Dependency

O Lord, hear my prayer,
Listen to my cry for mercy;
In your faithfulness and righteousness
Come to my relief. (Psalm 143:1)

Christmas was over and life resumed back to its normal routine. My pain and stiffness continued to worsen and now all of my joints ached. Dr. Thomson had no explanation for my pain and I was becoming more and more concerned. I suspected I had bone cancer. Oh God, I am so scared something is seriously wrong with me again! ***"O Lord, heal me, for my bones are in agony." (Psalm 6:2).*** Why else would I have constant pain? The only thing that helped ease the pain was the Oxycotin and Oxycodone. As time passed I needed more painkillers and the pain only increased. I became very scared about my condition, as did Dr. Thomson.

I was seeing him at least once a week about my pain and felt embarrassed and uncomfortable asking for more painkillers. The truth of the matter was I was more than just accustomed to them; I was actually dependent on them. Of course I took them for the pain, but I must admit I also took them for the sense of well being they gave me. So began a vicious circle in more than one way. First, in order to obtain the good feelings I experienced from the pills I had to take more and more in order to reach the same level of "contentment". Second, I would have to take more and more pills to ease the pain and discomfort in my bones. I realized I had a problem with painkillers and I knew my body was physically addicted to them. To stop taking them would mean experiencing detox again. Oh hell! I didn't want to go through that "hell on earth" again, and I enjoyed the pills too much to stop. I refused to give them up. That meant I had to continue to see the doctor to get more painkillers even though I felt terribly embarrassed about doing so.

I found myself at the doctor's office many, many times anxiously waiting for a prescription for painkillers. Dr. Thomson hated giving me the pills and was extremely concerned about it. He knew full well I had become dependent on them, but nothing else helped ease my pain. One morning while speaking to Dr. Thomson he told me he suspected my pain was caused by the painkillers. That was something I didn't want to hear even though I wanted the pain to go away in the worst way. Oxycotin and Oxycodone can cause rebound pain. It made perfect sense. That explained why no other pain medication worked and also explained why my pain was always getting worse. When I returned home I flushed a half bottle of Oxycotin down the toilet. There! Now let's see if my pain gets better. I still had Oxycodone of course! Two days later my pain was considerably better, but I was getting dangerously low on Oxycodone. Back to see Dr. Thomson.

When I got to the doctor's office I was disappointed to learn Dr. Thomson was not in his office that day. I was able to see a different doctor. I explained to him how I had flushed my pills down the toilet and how much better I was . This doctor was very pleased and knew Dr. Thomson would be too. I worked up the courage to ask for another prescription of Oxycodone and he was happy to give me one. Fantastic! I could go home feeling so much better physically and enjoy my painkillers. I was even happier when I seen how many pills he had prescribed - lots. Plenty to enjoy for the next two weeks. This cycle continued for the next two months. I knew this could not continue much longer and I dreaded the day I would be forced to quit taking my pills.

One morning in early February this problem came to a head. I had been getting low on my pills, so I was forced to cut back considerably. I was no longer getting large quantities from the doctor. He was trying so hard to wean me off of these things, much to my disappointment. I had woken up feeling the first symptoms of drug withdrawal. I immediately took the last of my painkillers and still could feel drug withdrawals. I was very scared to go through detox and very scared to ask Dr. Thomson for more pills. The withdrawals were getting worse. Oh God, what a horrible feeling. Physically my body was demanding more painkillers and mentally I would do what I had to in order to get them. Randal had left for work and I sat in my "God room" crying and praying. Oh God help me out of this mess! As my body suffered the "heebie jeebies" of detox again I knew what I had to do. I had to go out into that cold winter morning and ask Dr. Thomson for more pills. I cried at the thought because I hated having to do this.

As I sat and waited for Dr. Thomson, I wished he was away and I could see a different doctor. It was always so much easier to get the painkillers from the other doctors. I was a cancer patient and they wanted to take care of me, unaware I had a real problem with these drugs. One of the doctors was about to write me a prescription one afternoon and then she saw a note on my file, "Under no circumstance is any physician to prescribe Oxycodone unless consulted by Dr. Thomson." This doctor consulted Dr. Thomson and I was not given the prescription. I felt so angry and embarrassed. I only had a few pills left and I had to return the next day to ask Dr. Thomson for the prescription. He reluctantly gave me a small prescription. This morning I knew he would not want to give me any more pills. I nervously waited for him.

Dr. Thomson came into the office and I once again explained I needed more painkillers. He reminded me how many I had taken in the past week. To deny this, or to attempt to lie about it would have been silly. I would have made a fool of myself, so I had no other choice but to admit to it. I could easily see Dr. Thomson was not happy with me. I could see he wanted to scold me, and he would have had every right to do so. Reluctantly he wrote me a small prescription and told me exactly what he was thinking, "Don't take more than what is prescribed." I left my doctor's office that morning feeling terribly embarrassed and somewhat ashamed. However, I also felt so happy knowing the heebie jeebies would soon disappear and I would be feeling fine in a short period of time.

How did I get to this point? All my life I had been so sensible when it came to drugs and alcohol. Sure, I drank some and smoked some pot when I was young, but never did I try anything stronger. I always believed drugs were a dead end and had known people that had allowed drugs to ruin their lives. I would love to say I was far too intelligent to do drugs, but truthfully I was just too scared. If anyone would have ever told me I would experience drug withdrawals I would have thought they were crazy. I was so positive that was something I would never have to go through.

Now here I sat, knowing I could not continue like this much longer and terrified of detox. "Oh God, get me out of this mess!"

I had finished this prescription in record time. It only took me one day to take the 15 pills I had been given. I was again very scared about going through detox and very embarrassed and afraid to see Dr. Thomson to ask for more. The jig was up. I had to go see my doctor and admit to him I had a real problem with painkillers. I sure didn't want to do this, but I had no other options. Once again I nervously sat in my doctor's office to ask for more pills. I hated this so very much. Dr. Thomson entered the room with his usual smiling face and pleasantly asked what he could do for me. I immediately broke down and admitted my problem. He of course had already known this, and I'm sure he was pleased to see me finally admitting it to myself. He wrote me out a prescription for 5 lousy little pills. Oh no! How the hell was I going to avoid detox with 5 little pills?

Feeling defeated, I went to the pharmacy to have this prescription filled. As I stood at the counter waiting for assistance I took a black pen and placed a number one in front of the five. I was relieved nobody saw me do this and had very high hopes of this scheme working. It didn't work. I returned home with tremendous disappointment and fear knowing I would be going into drug withdrawals very soon. At that minute I decided no matter how horrible I felt I would not go to Dr. Thomson for more pills. The worst of the detox would occur during the weekend, and that would allow me the time I needed to avoid a trip to Dr. Thomson's office. I was now determined the time had come to put an end to this craziness.

My withdrawals began that evening. I admitted to Randal what was happening and he assured me he would help me through the days to come. I was relieved I did not have to suffer through this alone, but frightened by the physical horror I would not be able to escape from. I did not sleep one wink that night. I was wide awake all night long. That horrible sensation throughout my body was horrendous. I prayed God would ease the sensation, but no such luck. This detox was not as severe as the first time. I was able to lay still instead of moving constantly, which was a great relief to me. I was very lucky to not experience any nausea, however I had terrible diarrhea. Randal slept on the couch that night, so I had the bedroom all to myself. I tried to watch a movie on television. It was a mob story, but I was unable to enjoy it. Normally, I love mob movies, and I had seen this movie before. However, this night the violence really bothered me. I found it very gory and very disturbing. Besides, it was hard to pay attention because I had too many "heebie jeebies".

I heard Randal downstairs at 6:00 am. I joined him in the kitchen and told him about my night. We both hoped I would be able to get some sleep during the day, but were doubtful. I didn't get any sleep that day, and spent the entire day trying to get comfortable and going to the toilet. I have much more sympathy for drug addicts now. I understand better what they experience, and pray for them to get better.

Night eventually came and I didn't sleep one wink again. I was so exhausted. I sat on my bed battling the "heebie jeebies", the waves of body heat and the chills, and rocking back and forth. The rocking helped ease the "heebie jeebies" and at times I almost fell asleep. It was another long night. This process would be so much easier if one could sleep it off. I thought of many things. I thought a lot about God and the universe and Heaven and on and on and on. I spent a considerable amount of time thinking about the Holocaust. How could God allow such horrors to occur? I blame the drug withdrawals for the numerous negative thoughts I had. Oh God help me get over this as quickly as possible.

Morning came and I was very tired. All I wanted to do was sleep. I continued to lie in my bed feeling the "heebie jeebies". I begged God to be with me and help me. I became very worried my detox would get worse and this really scared me, *"Do not hide your face from me or I will go down to the pit."* *(Psalm 143:7)* I was already in a pit and desperately wanted out. I remembered the promise Jesus made about rest, *"Come to me, all you who are weary and burdened, and I will give you rest..." (Matthew 11:28)* I reminded God of this promise, and prayed that morning for rest. I was able to sleep for two hours that morning.

I had a dream that broke my heart, but strengthened my determination. In my dream I was healthy. I was wearing a pink hooded pullover, white shorts, white socks and white sneakers. My hair was long enough to have a ponytail. I was the slim shapely woman I had once been, and I was happy. I had so much energy and was running in a neighbourhood I lived in years ago. In the dream I felt wonderful being healthy again and being a reflection of what I had once looked like. When I woke up I cried. I was so sad and disappointed it was only a dream. I was still chubby with very short dark hair, still undergoing cancer treatment, and still experiencing drug withdrawals. I made a promise to myself that morning - I would one day be that woman in my dream, but for now I had to accept the situation I was in.

It was day four of the drug withdrawals and I was not feeling any better. I had only slept those two hours. My body was exhausted, but my mind was very much alert. I laid in my bed feeling horrible, wishing I could only sleep. I was able to fall asleep for an hour, and I had a very disturbing dream. This dream was violent and terrifying. I was alone in downtown Fort St. John. There was snow and ice on the ground, and it was very cold. It was night and I had to sleep in the street. I huddled into an alcove, covered myself up with a blanket, and shivered as I tried to fall asleep. As I lay there I was terrified someone was going to stab me. My friend Joanna had told me someone was going to kill me that night and told me I had to be careful. I pulled the blanket over my head and peeked out making sure no one was coming towards me. In my mind I was planning an escape route. As my mind raced, I was angry at Joanna for not letting me stay at her house and angry at Randal for not letting me in the house. Weird! I found a ruler with a metal edge and if anyone came I was going to stab them with it. I survived the night and in the morning I left to go home. I was in the same neighbourhood as in the previous dream. I made it home alive and then I woke up. I knew the strange dreams were due to the drug withdrawal, and hoped they would end soon.

Later that day I went to see Dr. Thomson. I so wanted him to give me a prescription for Oxycodone, but I didn't ask and he didn't offer. I asked if I could get something to help me sleep, but he told me nothing would help. He explained my sleep pattern would go back to normal in a few days. A few days seemed like a very long period of time. However, he did give me a few Valium to help me with my anxiety. Thank you Dr. Thomson! You have no idea how much I appreciated that! I was finally able to get a few hours of sleep that night.

By day seven of detox the withdrawals had lessened considerably, but were still bothersome. I was still feeling the "heebie jeebies", still feeling hot and cold, and still not sleeping much. I feared this would never end! I lay on my bedroom floor attempting to relieve my discomfort, and prayed God would let this end soon. I must have prayed about 20 minutes and then made my way downstairs. As I was coming down the staircase I stopped and prayed. I then noticed the "heebie jeebies" were gone. Finally they were gone! My body once again felt normal. What bliss! Seriously, what bliss! At the end of ten days all drug withdrawals had vanished and I was back to myself. No longer a slave to painkillers. Thank you God for helping me make it out of that hell.

I think it is important to remember all the people that are unfortunate enough to be a slave to a drug of any form. It is a horrible situation to be in. It seems to be a helpless and hopeless situation. I can better understand how a person can become addicted to drugs and I can better understand how hard it is to live addicted to drugs. It takes a person a great deal of courage to come clean and stay clean. God be with all of them! I had three months of treatment left and I honestly couldn't fathom it ever ending. I had to go without painkillers for my next treatment, but I was no longer dependent and that meant so much.

I Just Want My Health Back!

The Lord will sustain him on his sickbed
And restore him from his bed of illness. (Psalm 41:3)

I arrived at the hospital for my next treatment in the morning and everything occurred as usual until another woman walked into the room. She started speaking to Janice and Virginia. She was a loud boisterous person, and I found her presence to be intrusive. I was now a veteran at this chemo department and I had a feeling of ownership. I felt very possessive of Janice and Virginia; they were my nurses. I felt the same way about Dr. Thomson - he was my doctor. This woman roared into the chemo room and loudly rattled on about herself. Yuck! I so did not want to listen to this woman's story. She had just started her treatment and had come into see Janice and Virginia to show them her bald head. Wow! Like she was the only person who has lost her hair! I felt contempt for this woman. She continued to roar with descriptions of her sex life. Oh God! Sex - what a horrible thought.

Randal and I had not had sex in months. I had been far too sick and I had gone into menopause giving me a very dead libido. Sex was not an issue in my life, so to be forced to endure this woman's concerns regarding her sex life made me want to vomit. Yuck! I didn't care if she and her husband still had great sex! I didn't care when she said how worried she was about getting pregnant! Really, this woman was new at this cancer thing. I guess no one told her she would not be able to get pregnant. At least that is what I had been told. Due to my hysterectomy, that had not

141

been an issue for me, but I didn't feel the need to let everyone know about it. She continued on revealing that she had been using a diaphragm. Way too much information! In my mind I saw this obese woman inserting her diaphragm. Yuck! By now I felt disgust for this woman and wished she would just leave. But no, she had to start on about her nausea.

Was it just me or does hardly anyone take their anti-nausea drugs? This woman didn't. Smart! She roared on about how much nausea she suffered from, but didn't want to take anything for it believing she was physically strong enough that the nausea would disappear. That was one of the dumbest things I have ever heard. What did she think Janice and Virginia were going to think? "Wow Lady, are you ever a brave woman!" Clearly this woman was new to the game. I wanted to tell her how unimpressed I was. Instead of feeling compassion, I thought to myself, "Just wait lady, your little positive attitude will disappear just like mine did." Yes, my attitude had become bitter and I no longer had the oxycodone to give me a sense of well being.

It was only later I was able to understand my attitude towards this woman. My disgust was never really towards her, it was towards myself. I was very resentful I had lost my positive attitude, sense of adventure, and fighting spirit. I was resentful I had become exhausted, frustrated, and sick and tired of being sick and tired. I was bitter about all the things cancer had taken away from me. I was bitter because I had lost myself on so many levels. I was disappointed in myself for not maintaining a wonderful attitude to the bitter end. I had thought I would be a better patient. I was sad all the time. I did not feel like a survivor, but more of a zombie - the walking dead. I sank into another deep depression, one that would take me months to get out of.

It was late February and still winter in northern Canada. This added to my depression, but then it seemed everything added to my depression. I was depressed I was still in treatment, depressed about my weight gain, depressed about my appearance, depressed about my poor health, and jealous of everyone else for being healthy. Ever since I had that dream where I was happy and healthy again, I couldn't stop thinking about it. I longed more than words can describe for that dream to be my reality, but it wasn't. What could I do to help myself? I had become consumed by depression and I didn't know how to help myself. I kept this struggle to myself until I could no longer hold it in.

It was at this time I noticed my eyesight becoming increasingly worse, especially my right eye. One afternoon while my mom was visiting me I told her about my eyes. As she listened I became more and more upset. I went into the kitchen and began to cry. I sat down on the floor and sobbed. I was overcome by sadness. I bellowed out, "All I want is my health back! I just want my body back again! Everything is breaking down! I can't even see right anymore! People don't know how lucky they are when they have their health! When you don't have your health, you have nothing!" My mom reassured me that I would have my health back one day, but I bellowed out, "You don't know that! I'll never be healthy again!" Despite my emotional state I was able to search the phone book and make an appointment with an optometrist for the following week. Times were so dismal for me, its hard to believe they were only going to get worse.

I went to the hospital for my next treatment with great resentment. When I walked into the chemo room I was instantly angry. There was a patient in every recliner, and I had hoped there would be nobody there. My thoughts and desires were becoming more and more self-centered, but I didn't care. Janice pleasantly explained they were running late and would soon have a recliner for me. I understood of course, but I was still ticked off I had to wait. I took a pamphlet from the bookcase and began to read it. The pamphlet described many emotions patients experience when nearing the end of their treatment. I was relieved to learn many cancer patients feel the same way I was feeling. I learned the sadness I was feeling was actually grief. I was grieving the loss of my health. Up to this point I had been rather positive about my situation, and had become discouraged by my depression. Yes, I miss being healthy. I miss not having to worry about my health. I miss not wondering what next is going to break down on my body. I miss not being jealous of others for their good health. As I continued to read I could feel myself getting very close to crying. I didn't want to cry in front of everyone, so I went into the bathroom and tried to cry as quietly as possible. I remained in the bathroom crying for what seemed to be ten minutes. When I came out I was happy to see a recliner waiting for me.

I sat myself down and waited for either Janice or Virginia to begin the process of plugging me in to that horrible I.V.. When Janice began the process, she asked, "How is your chest?" I thought that was a very strange question - one I had not yet heard. "Fine. Why?" Janice's reply surprised me, "I thought I heard you wheezing in the bathroom." Oh Shit! They could hear me! I was too sad to feel embarrassed, so I told Janice and Virginia, "I was just having a good cry." I barely had the words out of my mouth and I began to cry again. I believe this was the first time both nurses had seen me cry. I had wanted to be brave, but now that notion was shot. Janice and Virginia reacted with great care and concern. I felt very fortunate to have such wonderful nurses I could turn to. I let it all out. I told them everything. Janice pulled up joke on the computer, attempting to cheer me up. Virginia showed me a picture of her and Janice doing yoga together. I told them how much I wanted to do yoga, and cried because I was still too sick to do much. They were so understanding, and reassured me I would get better one day. Janice asked me if I kept a journal and for the first time I told someone outside of my family that I was writing a book. They seemed really delighted and gave me their permission to use their real names. We spoke all about my book. I told them almost everything I was writing, and when the subject of spirituality arose I shared some of my experiences with them. I described the cocoon of protection I felt and much to my delight they told me they have heard the same thing from other cancer patients. Janice had to attend to another patient, but Virginia and I continued to talk about God.

Virginia told me she was a believer too, but didn't go to church on a regular basis. I don't either. So what? I told Virginia she goes to church every day she works. Isn't that what church is? I don't believe going to a building every Sunday is going to church. That is not to say I don't believe people should do that - they should if that is what they wish to do. I believe going to church is sharing God's love with others no matter what day it is, or where it takes place. That way people can go to church whenever they want and as often as they want. Just think about it - don't most significant "religious experiences" occur outside of church? Mine do. People are in church every day without even realizing it! Nothing irritates me more than the abuse of religion. So many horrible things have happened in the world in the name of religion.

What is religion? I believe Mark 7:6-7 describes religion very accurately, ***"These people honour me with their lips, but their hearts are far from me. They worship me in vain; their teachings are but rules taught by men."*** Is it not religion that turns a blind eye to the molestation of innocent children? Is it not religion that has forced women and children to remain with abusive husbands and fathers. Is it not religion that turns millions of human beings away based on marital status, gender, colour, and sexuality? Is it not religion that preaches that the good and deserving are married men and women with their own children? Is it not religion that states people that follow the rules will go to Heaven even if they are hypocrites ignoring Galatians 2:21? ***"I do not set aside the grace of God, for if righteousness***

could be gained through the law, Christ died for nothing!" If religion could be taken out of the church, church would be a great place for all believers to attend.

Before leaving the hospital that day I made sure I told Virginia just how important she and Janice are, and how important their jobs are. True heroes are not on a big screen. They are in all corners of the world - doing the good the world doesn't always see. I left the hospital - or should I say "church" that day feeling so much better. It was comforting to be able to share so much with Janice and Virginia.

After the hospital I went for my eye appointment. I was told I had cataracts in both eyes, but my right eye was especially bad. I was also told I would have a rather long wait before I could get the corrective surgery. This doctor referred me to every hospital in our area and I hoped the wait would not be too long. I was both disappointed and relieved about my eyes. There was nothing seriously wrong with my eyes and the condition could be fixed permanently. The biggest drag about my eyes was I could no longer drive. Another thing cancer robbed me of.

Later when Randal came home from work I told him about my eyes, and my experience at the hospital. I explained to him how I was grieving the loss of my health and I once again cried. I told Randal how I felt my illness had made an old woman out of me. I continued to cry as I revealed all my feelings to him. Then he said something really stupid and insensitive, "You're not the only person to go through this." I couldn't believe what I heard! What was he trying to say? Was he trying to tell me to "Shut up and quit whining. Other people go through this too and don't cry about it. You don't have it any rougher than anyone else, now get over it." I told him what a thoughtless thing that was to say to me, and within five minutes he was snoring on the couch. I was furious! As he lay snoring I packed a change of clothes and phoned Nick to come and pick me up. I spent the night crying about it to my mom. I didn't go home the next day until I got an apology. Randal and I were able to discuss everything and he was much more understanding.

I had started to read a book I brought home from the hospital with me the previous day called, "Living Beyond Breast Cancer", written by Marisa C. Weiss, M.D. and Ellen Weiss. I recommend this book to all breast cancer survivors. It is an excellent source of information that is much needed. I had thought my mental health would begin to improve as I got closer to the end of my treatment. I was astonished when this didn't happen. It wasn't until I started reading this book that I was able to understand why I was feeling the way I was. It all made perfect sense! I learned that the seriousness of my cancer didn't hit me until all the "excitement," or "busyness," or whatever one wishes to call it was over. With most of the treatment behind me I was now able to feel the strong emotions of horror, terror, heartbreak, and grief I had been too shocked to feel before. Now was the time to begin healing my spirit and I knew this was possible with God's help and my own will to overcome. I just didn't realize how much worse my situation would become.

I am not a patient woman and I grow frustrated when I do not make as much progress as I expect. Lack of progress deepened my depression and by March it seemed no one could help me. Dr. Thomson referred me to Dr. Joyce Smith, a psychiatrist. My first appointment with her would be in May. Never in my life did I ever think I would have to see a psychiatrist. I have no shame about it though. Actually I am glad to tell others I am under the care of a psychiatrist because it proves I am willing to do whatever I have to in order to get better physically and mentally. Besides, Dr. Smith is a wonderful lady and she is a cat lover too!

I went to the hospital for my treatment and felt deeply bitter I had to be there. Janice was not working that day, but Virginia was her usual happy self. There was a new addition to the chemo room - a T.V.. Virginia put a funny movie on for me while I took my treatment. That was a nice gesture and I was able to forget most of my problems. However, I could still feel resentment about having to be there. I was also becoming very anxious about my vision, and had a difficult time trying not to think about it.

March was uneventful, however Randal and I travelled to Alberta to see an eye surgeon. He told me my cataracts were white. I didn't realize they came in colors. That explained why my vision was a blurry white instead of darkening vision. The surgeon also confirmed the steroids had caused the cataracts. After meeting with the surgeon, as I was walking back to the truck, the wind blew. That was the first time I felt the wind blow through my hair since I lost it. What a wonderful sensation! I would only have to wait six to eight weeks for my surgery. Thank God, as I was growing more and more anxious about my vision. This anxiety was becoming serious, and my mental state was deteriorating without me realizing just how much. I had to keep it together somehow, but how?

My mother decided to move back to Vancouver Island in June, so she temporarily moved into my house in April. Everything was going okay. I was still going to the hospital every three weeks for my treatment, and I was still experiencing pain and stiffness in my knees. I had not taken the

Oxycodone since the end of February, so Dr. Thomson had prescribed steroids to help with the pain. These steroids aggravated the cataracts, and I did notice a remarkable decline in my eyes after each treatment. My right eye became much worse after my treatment in April.

My birthday was approaching and I wanted to get a tattoo on my lower leg above my ankle. I had drawn a picture of a pink ribbon wrapped around a cross, and added the date of my diagnosis to it. This tattoo signified my illness in the form of the pink ribbon and signified how I got through each day by the addition of the cross. On April 23rd, the afternoon of my birthday, Joanna drove me down to the tattoo parlour. The tattooist had a great sense of humour. He made me feel very comfortable, erasing all nervousness I was feeling.

Just as he was about to begin working, a woman entered the shop. She was a slim beautiful woman about my age. I immediately felt very jealous of her. Oh God, why do I have to be me? I was so envious of her beauty and felt so embarrassed by my own appearance. I had taken a considerable amount of time getting ready for this appointment and all my efforts were for nothing. I looked like shit. I not only felt jealous, I felt inferior to her. All my looks had been ravished by chemotherapy. I felt so sure this woman would go home and tell her family about the ugly fat lady getting a tattoo. I so wanted to explain to her why I was so ugly. Earlier in my treatment this would not have bothered me. I would have just felt gratitude about being alive. Deep bitterness had taken root into my spirit, and I didn't know what to do about it. At this point I decided to quit dwelling on this woman and concentrate on my tattoo.

I had never been a tattoo person. I had always thought they were ugly and could never understand why anyone would want to mark up their body in such a gaudy fashion, but here I lay getting one myself. To hell with what other people think! This was important to me. My tattoo was a badge of courage I could look at anytime I needed to in order to remind myself of how far I have come. I was proud of it and wanted the world to see it. It didn't even hurt!

Randal gave me a wonderful birthday party that evening. He brought home a couple of large pizzas, a huge birthday cake and invited all the kids. It felt good to have everyone I loved around me. Although I was turning 45, I was happy to celebrate another birthday! I was still alive! I was so thankful to God for the gift of life and family! Too bad these happy feelings would not last long.

The following week I returned to the hospital for my treatment and proudly showed off my tattoo to Janice and Virginia. Apart from the good company, I felt very uncomfortable due to my right eye. It was as though I had something in it. Well I guess I did, but I could not remove this something, and it was very irritating. I had a big blind spot and much of what I could see was blurry. I could not concentrate on anything, because all I could think about was my lack of vision. A couple days later I had become completely blind in my right eye, and my vision was very poor in my left eye. Due to the extreme irritation I felt about the vision in my right eye I covered it up with a patch, but this did not help me much.

One afternoon I was sitting and talking with my mom about my eyes and a wave of horror came over my being. Suddenly I felt very panicky. I knew this was because of the loss of more than half of my eyesight. I was terrified I would never regain my vision. Oh God, please don't let me go blind! As much as the eye patch cured the blind spot in my right eye it caused me to experience a sense of being enclosed. Many times I wished I could just jump out of my body and be free. Each day dragged by as slow as the one before. Due to my lack of vision I did not feel like seeing others or going anywhere. Joanna would take me out on walks on sunny days to get me out of the house. As we walked and talked I thought about my eye constantly. I cannot explain how low I felt about my eyesight. I often wondered if I would be able to live if I did not regain my vision. During our walks I know I mentioned my vision frequently. Joanna told me a side effect of steroids is cataracts, "I didn't want to tell you that, because it is rare." My reply, "Oh, if it is rare I'll get it!" I was a different person - I didn't know who I was anymore. I prayed everyday I would not have to wait long for my surgery. Another problem - waiting.

While I was waiting to hear when my surgery date would be my family situation became unmanageable. Although Randal would not admit it, I know my illness had taken a toll on him. He had been supporting the family in every aspect for more than a year and I could see he was growing tired of this role. Melissa was pushing the boundaries that had been set for her and this caused enormous friction between her and Randal. I was unfortunately caught in the middle. Melissa did everything every other teenage girl does. Yes, she lied about where she was at times. Yes, she stayed out beyond her curfew. Yes, she skipped classes. Yes, she had become a worry to me and to Randal. I could handle this, but Randal could not. He became increasingly agitated by her, and with each wrong move she made, his stress increased. As Randal's stress increased so did mine, as he expected me to control her. How can a person control someone that is hell-bent on doing what they want?

I tried everything I could think of to get Melissa to comply with the house rules but nothing worked. She was failing all but one subject in school and Randal and I were both afraid she would end up dropping out of high school. I literally begged her to go to classes. At a complete loss, I phoned her father and he suggested Randal and I back off and then maybe she would improve on her own without our pressure. I could do this, but Randal could not. I told him repeatedly to back off and let her father and I handle the matter. The situation only grew worse.

Randal reached his breaking point on Mother's Day. Matthew and Nicholas came over to visit. Nick gave me a very pretty Mother's Day angel and Matthew was going to take me out for supper - just Matt and me. Before Matt and I left for the restaurant Randal, myself, Mom, Matt and Nick all visited together. Everything was fine until Randal started on about Melissa. He made a few unnecessary comments, but when he told me "… all she does is lie to you" I became angry, but calmly stated, "Actually Melissa and I have a great relationship." Randal laughed arrogantly and stated very bluntly, "That's because you believe all her bullshit." Now I was very angry and yelled, "Melissa and I have a close relationship!" Yes - AWKWARD. Randal quietly got up and went outside, while Matthew and I left for the restaurant.

When I returned home I quickly discovered my above comments were the last Randal could take. Randal sat me down and gave me an ultimatum, "I don't know what you're going to do, but you're going to have to leave." He gave me no opportunity to speak as he continued, "I'm not happy. The way you spoke to me in front of everyone was terrible. All I could do was leave the room to think about what to do." By this time Randal's face was red and his voice filled with hatred was elevating as he continued, "I've thought about this since you left and I'm not happy!" You are going to have to leave!" I sat in shock and was completely devastated. I was going to have to leave! I immediately enquired, "Where am I supposed to go? I'm not even finished treatment. I can't see and I can't drive. What do you think I am supposed to do?" Randal always has an answer, "You can go to the women's shelter. You can take your mother and your daughter with you. You won't be blind forever and once you get your eyes fixed you will be able to drive again." I reminded him that I no longer had a car to drive since my accident the day before I found out I had cancer and no longer had a job to support myself and my daughter. Again he had an answer, "Oh well, you will eventually get another car after you go back to work. Your treatment will be over soon and you'll just have to go back to work again and support yourself. All I know is I'm not happy!" I had become extremely angry and shouted back. "And I am?!" I wanted to throw a brick at his face. Randal ended the conversation by telling me I either get Melissa under control or she, my mother and I could move out. He told me to go up to my bedroom and not to tell my mother what was going on.

Feeling shocked, angry and devastated I did as I was told. I knew Randal meant every word he said and I didn't know what to do. I was being forced to chose between my husband and my daughter. How does a woman make such a choice? I was not emotionally or physically strong enough to handle this situation. I heard Randal go outside, so I went to my mom's room to talk to her about it. She could not believe it either. We sat together and tried to come up with some kind of solution, but were unable to do so.

My anxiety became very bad. I could not even be in the same room as Randal without having a panic attack. As soon as he came home from work I would start to sweat, shake and become very afraid. I felt frightened all the time. I prayed for strength and for answers. I prayed God would do something, so I wouldn't have to. If I was healthy like everyone else I could do something! Being as weak as I was I felt helpless to do anything. I was totally devastated!

As each day passed Melissa continued to skip classes and stay out past curfew on weekends. Randal's anxiety was worsening and he was pressuring me on a daily basis to fix her. Randal and I quit sleeping together months prior, and he made a habit of coming into our bedroom early in the morning and yelling at me about Melissa. He demanded to know where she was the night before, what time she came home, if she worked after school, did she get her pay check. Randal had come to the point that he felt he had to have complete control over every aspect of my daughter's life. He also came to believe I had to support his every unreasonable action he took against my daughter. I now realized - truly realized Randal hated me and my children.

One day at the end of May, Randal demanded I tell Melissa she was no longer allowed to live in our home (her home). He demanded I tell her to "get the fuck out." I was sick with confusion and felt completely helpless. How could I ever kick my daughter out of my house? That beautiful baby girl I prayed so much for, how? She was God's most precious gift and Randal was tossing her out of my house like a piece of garbage. I refused to deal with it the way Randal demanded, so I asked Nicholas and Matthew if she could live with them for the rest of the school year until she went to stay with her father for the summer. They agreed. It would have gone smoothly if it were not for Randal.

Just because it was not Randal's idea Melissa live at her brother's home he decided it was a bad idea. He said, "No. No way." He demanded I come up with a different plan - his plan. He demanded I phone her father and tell him she was going to be coming to live with them as soon as possible. Melissa's dad was shocked by what I was telling him. I explained how Randal had become out of control and how he was picking on our daughter. Her father did not realize the magnitude of Randal's demands and agreed he would take her at the end of the school year. Randal was furious. It was only a couple days later he forced me to tell Melissa to get out of the house. He yelled at me, "I don't care where she goes just as long as she gets the fuck out of here!" I was devastated. Being absolutely terrified I went to Melissa's bedroom and told her she had to go to her brother's home. This was a nightmare! She agreed to live with her brothers, but she really had no other choice. How can someone be so cruel to a young girl?

Matthew was helping Melissa to pack up some of her belongings when Randal arrived home just in time to cause a whole lot of trouble. Randal began watching every move Melissa and Matthew made. I was sitting on the back porch as Melissa and Matthew started loading her things into Randal's truck that he had so kindly let them borrow. Randal made sure he was there too, listening to every word and interjecting with his arrogant sarcasm. Oh how I wished I could kill him. I thought he was a monster. A real man doesn't do this to a young girl. A real man doesn't abuse his family. All too soon Melissa and Matt were ready to pull away and I stood and cried as I watched them leave. They were gone about 15 minutes when Randal became alarmed the kids hadn't returned his truck yet. What a bully! How long did he think it takes to move?

That was it for me right then. I yelled at Randal to shut up. I phoned Matthew and asked him nicely to return the truck as soon as they are finished. "Well of course." Matt replied with disdain. When Matt and Melissa returned I told them I would be the next one Randal tosses out. My heart was broken. I could not believe this was happening. My daughter was gone from my home and I was helpless to do anything.

The morning after Melissa was gone I woke up feeling a great sense of fear. I didn't know what to do about this or my profound sense of sadness. My mom was in the kitchen when I came downstairs that morning and asked me how I was feeling. I told her how horrible I felt about the situation and she could see how torn up I was about it. It was this morning that I would have the worst experience of my life.

As I shared my feelings with my mom she tried to comfort me the best she could. I was in the bathroom crying when she came into see if she could help. All I could do was cry. I told my mom how I had lost everything. I had lost my breast, my health, my vision, my body, my looks, my independence, my marriage, and now my daughter. I cried uncontrollably as I yelled out, "I have nothing! I have lost everything!" My mom tried so hard to calm me down and reassure me my life would get better, but I just kept crying. My mom became very worried because she could see I was losing control of myself. Within minutes I was lying on the bathroom floor unable to stop crying. Within minutes of that I was screaming at the top of my lungs, "I have nothing!" And within minutes of that I was just screaming as loud as I could. I felt as though something terrible was about to happen - like I would die, or go crazy. I was gripped by total fear and the only way I could relieve this was to scream.

As I lay on the bathroom floor screaming out repeatedly, my mom became desperate to help me. She didn't know what to do. She begged me to let her phone an ambulance, but I refused as I screamed out, "No! If you do I will leave!" She then begged me to let her phone Dr. Thomson, but I again refused as I screamed out, "No! No way! He can't do anything to help me!" Mom tried to assure me Dr. Thomson would help, but I continued to refuse and continued to scream. My poor mother. She was so scared and didn't know how to convince me to get medical help. She insisted I let her phone 911, but all I could do was scream. As my mom begged me to get help I tried to hide in an unfinished closet in the bathroom, but knowing I could not hide I laid on the bathroom floor screaming. Finally my mom said, "If you don't let me phone Dr. Thomson I am going to phone 911." I realized she was serious and being terrified the ambulance would come I did not argue with her and she made the call.

I could faintly hear my mom on the phone in the kitchen as I lay on the bathroom floor screaming over and over as loud as I could. I had a feeling of impending disaster or death. I was positive I was about to die. I have never experienced such formidable fear in all my life. I screamed out to God, "Help me! Do something!" When my mom was finished on the phone she came into the bathroom. I looked at her and screamed, "God hates me! He has left me! I have nothing! I have lost everything!" Again my mom tried to comfort me. As I screamed she told me the nurse from Dr.

Thomson's office was coming to the house with some Valium. My mom urged me to try to calm down, but I just kept screaming. My mom has told me this carried on for at least 30 minutes, and then I slowly began to calm down. When I was able to stop screaming I asked my mom in desperation if she was telling me the truth about the nurse coming to the house. I was astonished someone cared. I was able to stop screaming, but could not stop crying uncontrollably. My mom helped me to my bedroom and waited with me for the nurse.

I lay on my bed breathing deeply and praying the nurse would arrive quickly. I still felt an incredible sense of impending doom and concentrated on remaining calm. While Mom and I were in my bedroom Matthew showed up. I didn't want him to see me that way. I became panicky again and started to cry. I said to Mom, "I don't want him to see me. He can't see me like this!" I got up from my bed and went and hid in my closet. My mom tried to calm me down and was deeply disturbed by my behaviour. She told me I didn't have to see Matthew. She said she would get rid of him. When she went downstairs I continued to hide in my closet feeling terrified something horrible was about to happen, and terrified Matthew would come upstairs and see me. Oh God, what will happen if Matthew comes up here? He didn't. The nurse arrived with the Valium just before lunch. I took two right away and Mom stayed with me until I felt better.

Once I had calmed down I looked at my mom and felt terrible for what she witnessed her daughter go through. I said to her, "That must be what a nervous breakdown feels like." She looked back at me and quietly said, "That was a nervous breakdown." She asked me how I felt and I was relieved to tell her I felt better. Despite everything I had been through in my life that was the worst day of my life. What a terrifying experience! I had lost all control and was so sure I was going to die. I felt like a sitting duck. I believed something horrible was going to come down on me at any second and God was nowhere. Oh God, what next? God, please just let me have my health back!

Melissa had come to see me one morning a couple of days after she left. I was in bed still very shaken from my breakdown. My cats were resting with me on the bed when she came into my room. I was so happy to see her, but still so very heartbroken over her and terrible feelings of guilt. As we talked she petted the cats and said, "Maybe one day we will all be reunited." Oh God, how my heart broke! All I wanted was to hold her and never let go. I prayed God would reunite us as she and I wanted so badly. I cried so hard when she left.

Anxiety and Panic Disorder

Answer me quickly, O Lord;
My spirit fails.
Do not hide your face from me
Or I will be like those who go down
To the pit.
Let the morning bring me word of
Your unfailing love. (Psalm 143:7-8)

That experience left me feeling terrified I would have another nervous breakdown. Randal was no help. When mom told him how upset I was he said, "That's easy enough to fix. Just slap her across the face next time." Every morning when I woke up I immediately felt fear. My stomach was extremely nervous. I had diarrhea throughout each day, my body temperature fluctuated between hot and cold, I would sweat uncontrollably, I would shake all over at times, I couldn't eat, I felt frightened frequently throughout the days, I would wrestle with thoughts of death and doom, and I had to remain in my bedroom most of the day trying to remain calm. No one could help me through this, certainly not my husband, not my kids, not my mom, not my friends, not Janice and Virginia, and not Dr. Thomson either. This was between God and me and only He could help me through this. I prayed for hours at a time trusting fully God would know what I was really needing, **"...the Spirit helps us in our weakness. We do not know what we ought to pray for, but the Spirit himself intercedes for us with groans that words cannot express. And He who searches our**

hearts knows the mind of the Spirit, because the Spirit intercedes for the saints in accordance with God's will." (Romans 8:26).

I was literally living on a prayer. I could not imagine my life beyond each day. I had lost all hope. I was certain something terrible would happen to me. I had never been as spiritually devastated in my life as I now was. I even doubted God would be able to help me. I shared my fears with my mom. I kept telling her everyday my life was finished -truly finished. She tried to convince me otherwise, but I could not accept what she was trying to tell me. I can remember one day in particular. She came up to my room in the morning to see how I was feeling. I told her I had a great amount of anxiety. She said to me, "Just try to remain calm. Your life will not always be like this." I got out of my bed and began to pace the floor while breathing deeply in order to stay calm. I truly did not want my mom to witness me lose control again. I disagreed with her statement and she said, "It may not seem like it, but you have a wonderful life ahead of you." I threw myself onto my bed and cried out, "No I don't! My life is over!" Being afraid of losing control again, I had to snap myself back into a state of calm. With my mom's help, I was able to remain calm. This would be a challenge I would have to face on a daily basis.

I had to work at keeping my anxiety under control every day all day. Usually by the supper hour, my anxiety would lessen and I could relax some. In the evening, Randal and I would watch some T.V. together in the living room. I honestly couldn't stomach too much time with him. During this time, I would experience moments when I would feel panic. I would get hot and sweaty. My stomach would become nervous and I would begin to shake. Immediately I would feel fear. In order to remain calm I would go up to my bedroom and watch T.V. there, and let Randal watch his boring shows in the living room. Every night I would watch a program about a group of rich housewives. Ironically, this show made me feel so much better about my own life.

These women had no clue of what life is about. They were so proud of themselves for marrying rich men and having all the material goodies they could get their hands on. They were so proud of their fake boobs, fake hair, heck - fake everything! Whenever I would listen to what these women said and did, I had to laugh to myself. One of the housewives was about to get a new set of boobs, "Very important in this community." she stated. Wow! All I wanted was an operation to regain my vision, "Very important in any community!" I would say. I would much rather have my vision than a great set of fake boobs. What I found the most entertaining about these women was their attitudes about helping those less fortunate. One woman in particular stated she felt no shame being rich and that it's important to help the poor. Wow! Really? What a saint! I wondered if she would have the same glib attitude if she was the poor one. I admit there were moments I envied these women, but by the end of the program, I was glad to be me. They could keep their empty lives. As scripture teaches the rich have their reward.

I truly believe I have so much more than those women have. Certainly, they have big beautiful houses, nice expensive cars, jewellery adorning their wonderfully plastic sculpted bodies, beautiful expensive clothes and so much more. But I have an inner peace about my death and destiny, despite my anxiety and panic. I am thankful for each day I am able to live. (I truly appreciate my eyesight!) I have an appreciation for my body, and know it is more important to have a healthy body than a perfect body. I have a healthy brain, and I can function independently within society. All my limbs work as they are supposed to. Yes, the rich have these too, but I truly know they are more precious than anything else in this world. I know the riches money can not buy, and thank God He has given them to me. I know what is important in this world. I am glad to have my faith and my health, because that is everything!

My good friend Juanita phoned me one afternoon. I saw her number on the call display and cringed when I saw it was her - not for any reason other than I did not want to talk to anyone. I took her call anyway and was very glad I did. I let her know just how dire my emotional state was and she gave me some very encouraging words. Juanita also reminded me that she and her husband lift my name up to God every Sunday during their church service. It felt so wonderful to have people help me even though I did not realize they were doing so. Juanita came by the house with some books about God, healing and comfort, a rosary, and a prayer book. All day in my bedroom I would pray and read the books. That was the only way I could remain calm. Thank God for Juanita! Thank you Juanita for your love, concern, and friendship.

I finally got the phone call about my eye surgery. I would have my operation June 1st I had a lot of fear about this operation, but then I had a lot of fear, period. I was afraid something would go wrong and I would be blind forever in my right eye. I was afraid I would lose control of myself on the operating table and have a panic attack. I was also afraid that once I arrived at the hospital I would be told I could not have the surgery for some stupid reason. All my fears were unfounded and I was able to have the operation without incident. I could not believe how smoothly everything went and I was astonished by how well I could see again. All the colours were so much more vibrant! What a gift! I felt so grateful to have my vision back in my right eye. People do not realize just how precious eyesight is. Now I do. There are so many times I am reminded of the loss of my vision. Every time I go for a walk, or drive, or read something. I no longer take it for granted and I thank God everyday for the precious gift of eyesight, and pray I never lose it again.

My mental health improved drastically after I had my surgery, but I still suffered from depression, anxiety and bouts of panic. While talking with Dr. Smith about my disorders I asked her what caused me to develop these conditions. She looked at me, smiled and said, "Wendy, you have experienced a great amount of losses in a very short period of time. You lost your breast, your health, your vision, your daughter. You lost your sense of well being. You have financial stress, marital stress; you are still going through treatment. It's no wonder you have depression and anxiety." I thought to myself, "Not to mention my weight gain and the loss of my looks." I had suffered numerous negative experiences within two years, which most people take a lifetime to experience. That being said, the time had come to regain my positive attitude I had lost.

At the end of the first week in June, I had to go to the hospital for my last treatment-Hooray! Before the big day, I went to see Dr. Thomson and he gladly gave me some Valium. Dr. Thomson was fully aware of my mental conditions and knew my treatments were a trigger for my anxiety. I was just relieved to have the Valium to get me through the first couple of days after my treatment. Feeling prepared for my last treatment Randal and I went to the hospital. When I walked into the chemo room, I saw two patients, and Janice and Virginia's smiling faces. I also noticed above one of the recliners some balloons and a sign reading, "Congratulations". I knew that was my seat, and was happy to take it. There was only one problem. This was not my last treatment.

I sat down in the recliner, Randal sat in a chair beside me and Janice pulled up a chair in front of me. I was still ignorant to my reality, but Janice enlightened me, "Wendy, Virginia says you have one more treatment after this one." I had suspected, but could not admit it to myself. I frowned at Janice's statement and she added, "Tell you what. We'll get you started on the I.V. and I will go into your file and count all your treatments to see if you do have another one left." I felt so disappointed and knew I really did have another one left to take. Janice returned later with the bad news and I told her and Randal I did not intend to take the last treatment. I was adamant this day would be the last day I would sit and take treatment. I was finished! Randal reminded me that I had declined the radiation and reminded me that I had agreed earlier in my treatment that I would complete all injections. Oh God, why did he have to remember that? I simply stated, "So?" I could tell he was leery to push me. At that point, Janice began to try to talk me into taking the last treatment. Suddenly I had a fantastic idea, "After this treatment I will wait until August and take the last one." Janice quickly replied, "Why?" Oh God, when will this nightmare ever end? I was so ready for this to be over, and so frustrated it was not. I was also frustrated with Janice and Randal. Why did they have to care this much? Why couldn't they just let this go? I told Janice I did not think one more treatment would make any difference. I was so sure she would not be able to argue with that reasoning, but "Studies have proven that 17 treatments of the Herceptin work. They used to give patients 20, but they found it made no difference. There is a very good reason why we give 17 treatments." Well shit! Being stubborn, I agreed to think about having the 17th treatment.

Like a reluctant trooper, I returned to the hospital three weeks later for the 17th and final treatment. It was about time! I felt no excitement. I only felt relief and resentment. My resentment was not directed at any one person. It was directed at my illness. I was terribly bitter about the condition of my life. I still believed I had lost everything. I was still deeply depressed and still suffering from panic attacks. I was suffering from empty nest syndrome and missing Melissa more than I thought possible. I could not even walk past her old bedroom without feeling an ache in my heart. Sometimes I would go into her old room, sit, and cry for her.

I felt so deeply saddened the day she flew down to Vancouver Island. I knew I was not emotionally strong enough to take her to the airport. Matthew brought her by before her flight so we could say our goodbyes. I cried hard as I held her tight, never wanting to let go. Oh how I wished the situation could be different. She left at 1:30 pm. When I knew her flight was leaving I went outside and watched for about a half an hour hoping to see her plane in the air. I never did. Oh please God, take care of my girl. Oh how I wished she were still in my home with me. I never told Janice or Virginia any of this. I did not want to burden them with my problems.

Janice and Virginia knew a few months prior I had reached my limit and knew there was nothing they could do to help me feel better.

One month after my final treatment I felt better physically and knew as time passed I would feel stronger. However, my mental health was still a huge issue. It was now when Joanna and I took another summer trip to Edmonton. Joanna was going to be moving to Washington State in a matter of weeks and had to get her passport. This time her son and daughter came with us on our trip. Joanna's kids are great kids. We had fun. Although the kids were with us all the time, Joanna and I still managed to get in some private talk -not much though. We had a great hotel room, but I had trouble with a man again! The hotel we were staying in had a restaurant. After checking in we all went to the restaurant for our supper. I had to go to the bathroom and once inside the little girl's room I chose a stall. I could see there was a woman in the stall next to mine, but I thought nothing of it. I did my business, stood up, pulled up my pants, and noticed through the crack between our stalls, this was no woman! There sitting on the toilet was a fat man. He was just sitting there doing nothing. I was unnerved and quickly got out of the stall. I noticed Joanna's 12-year-old daughter had come in and I waited for her to come out of the stall. As we washed our hands together, I whispered in her ear, "Hurry. There is a man in that stall just sitting there. Yes, she was surprised. I told a hotel worker when we left the bathroom. What is it about me and men whenever I go to Edmonton?

It was still a great couple of days. I really enjoyed my time with Joanna and her kids. Joanna is a special woman. I love listening to her speak because I enjoy her accent. She also has the cutest giggle and whenever I hear it, I feel good inside. Joanna phoned me routinely during my treatment and when I felt healthy enough she took me out of the house. She listened to all my complaints and was always understanding and patient. I could always depend on her if I needed something. Her kind heart and wonderful sense of humour always puts a smile on my face. She is a true friend and I cherish our friendship. I have watched Joanna evolve from a timid broken sparrow into a strong and independent woman. Thank you so very much, Joanna, for being with me during the worst days of my life!

Upon my return home from Edmonton, it was now the time to become a picture of health. That became my goal. I was determined to do whatever had to be done. I was looking forward to joining the Chronic Disease Management Program at the hospital. I was also looking forward to finally being off the steroids and being able to begin a diet plan. I knew that getting back to the woman I was three or four years ago was going to take a lot of hard work, but what a privilege! I had the privilege of working hard to become the woman I once was. With great confidence and knowing God is still with me working in my life I became very excited to begin a new chapter in my life - Life after Breast Cancer!

Epilogue

I will praise the Lord all my life;
I will sing praise to my God as long
As I live. (Psalm 146:2)

So much has changed in my life since my last treatment - too much to include in this book. As I write this I have been finished treatment for two years and I am working on my next book. Unfortunately I still suffer from Anxiety and Panic Disorder, but through medication it is under control. I am so very happy to mention my daughter's wish for us to be reunited has come to pass. After too many years of disappointment, misery and heartache my marriage ended. I moved from northern Canada to Vancouver Island and live with my mom, Melissa and our wonderful cats, Teddy and Mia. God is still in control of my life. He has delivered me from the pit of hopelessness and continues to bring comfort, hope and security into my life.

My pink ribbon journey has been the hardest thing I have had to endure in my life. However, I have become a richer woman because of it. My Christian faith has deepened and I am so grateful for what God has done for me. I sat at death's door terrified my life had come to an end. God not only washed away my fear of dying He gave me peace - letting me know I had more years to live. I have sensed a small portion of the peace and joy that waits for me one day. My belief in God is so much stronger than before. I know God is real - no one can ever convince me otherwise. I have felt God's presence and peace all around me and long to feel it again.

I will someday. God understands what it was like for me and so too does everyone else that has lived through cancer and treatment. In fact only those who have had cancer and treatment can truly understand how it feels. I have a bond with all survivors. We know.

We know how low we sank. We know how desperate we felt. We know the horror we had to face. We know what we had to do to get through each day. We know what it feels like to be a burden. We know how many tears we cried even though we lost count. We know how often we had to pray. We know how hard it is to hang in there. We know how frightening the future can be. We know the heartbreak of goodbyes. We know our darkest and deepest thoughts and fears. We know the profound sadness of losing our health. We know the profound sadness of being different. We know how cancer can isolate us from society. We know the heartbreak of cancer, but that is not all we know.

We know the joy of life. We know how precious life is. We know how precious our bodies and our health are. We know the importance of letting others know how much we love them. We know what is important in life - people! We know what is not important in life. We know each day is a triumph. We know who loves us. We know who we love. We know who and what real heroes are. We know our spirits. We know how strong we are. We know God and he knows us. We know each other's love, hope and understanding. We know how much life truly has to offer us. We know bullshit when we hear it! We know what is right and what is wrong. We know what is right for us and what is wrong for us. We know why it is important to fight for good. We know what good feels like. We know what love and faithfulness feels like. We know, truly know how short life is! We know there is more to life than T.V. We know how sick of T.V. we are! We know each other without knowing each other. We know we love each other. We know we are there praying for each other every day. God be with each one of you on your own pink ribbon journey and God bless all of you!

Acknowledgements

I humbly thank God above all others for His endless love, comfort, rest and support as He carried me through the most frightening experience of my life. I deeply thank my entire medical team! Special thanks to Dr. Mark Thomson for his kindness and patience - I know I was a rather demanding patient. Also my deepest gratitude to my nurses Janice and Virginia. Words cannot begin to express my appreciation for all your care and concern. Thanks to my mom - you have never failed to love and support me. You are my angel! Deepest thanks to my children, Nicholas - always there when I need you. Matthew - always my most curious supporter and Melissa - God's most precious gift! Warmest thanks to my best friends, Juanita and Joanna - your prayers and love helped me more than you will ever know. And finally, thank you Jann Arden for the gift of your music. Amen